MICHIGAN MAP K

D0252382

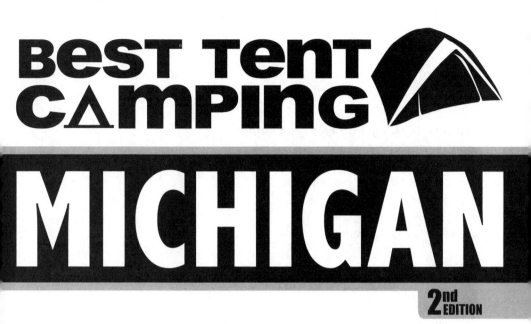

BEST TENT CAMPING

MICHIGAN

2nd EDITION

YOUR CAR-CAMPING GUIDE TO SCENIC BEAUTY, THE SOUNDS OF NATURE, AND AN ESCAPE FROM CIVILIZATION

MATT FORSTER

MENASHA RIDGE PRESS
Your Guide to the Outdoors Since 1982

:: *To all of the park rangers and volunteers who actually make our public lands work, and who must be doing it for love (it can't be the money). Thanks for sharing your stories with us.*

Best Tent Camping: Michigan, 2nd Edition
Copyright © 2015 by Matt Forster
All rights reserved
Printed in the United States of America
Published by Menasha Ridge Press
Distributed by Publishers Group West
Second edition, first printing

Library of Congress Cataloging-in-Publication Data

Forster, Matt, 1971–
  Best tent camping : Michigan : your car-camping guide to scenic beauty, the sounds of nature, and an escape from civilization / Matt Forster. — Second edition.
      pages cm
  "Distributed by Publishers Group West"—T.p. verso.
  Includes index.
  ISBN 978-1-63404-008-2 — ISBN 1-63404-008-2 — ISBN 978-1-63404-009-9 (eBook)
  1. Camping—Michigan—Guidebooks. 2. Camp sites, facilities, etc.—Michigan—Guidebooks. 3. Michigan—Guidebooks. I. Title.
  GV191.42.M5F67 2015
  917.74068—dc23

                                    2014047428

Cover design by Scott McGrew
Cover photo by Matt Forster
Text design by Annie Long
Maps by Steve Jones and Matt Forster
Indexing by Rich Carlson

Menasha Ridge Press
PO Box 43673
Birmingham, AL 35243
menasharidge.com

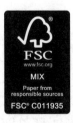

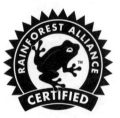

CONTENTS

● ●

BEST CAMPGROUNDS

● ●

ACKNOWLEDGMENTS

● ●

Many people contributed to this book with helpful information and by sharing some of their favorite places to camp. I first want to thank the hardworking people at the Michigan Department of Natural Resources (DNR) and the U.S. Forest Service. They do a bang-up job of providing the best campgrounds around.

There are well over a thousand campgrounds in this state, more than one person can fully appreciate. Numerous camping friends made sure their favorites weren't lost in the shuffle. They all shared their experiences of camping in Michigan and gave me productive suggestions. The folks who take time to post and respond on **Facebook.com/MichiganTent Camping** are always quick with suggestions and top-notch advice for campers.

Finally, I would like to thank you, the people who regularly leave home and live for a while in tents. By doing so, you support the state's campgrounds. Without a community of active and conscientious campers, outdoor recreation in Michigan wouldn't be the same. Keep camping, and I hope to see you out there!

—M. F.

PREFACE

● ●

I love camping in Michigan. Every campground here sits alongside some body of water—be it a river, stream, pond, or lake. (Perhaps it's the negative ions these waters generate that leave you feeling peaceful and relaxed after a week out in nature.) From grassy dunes overlooking Lake Michigan to thick woods along the Pine River to a quiet lake that serves as a portal to the Sylvania Wilderness, pitching a tent in Michigan opens the door to all sorts of adventure.

The largest state east of the Mississippi, Michigan is a land made for camping. Nowhere in the state are you ever farther than 85 miles from a Great Lake. With 36,000 miles of rivers and streams and 11,000 inland lakes, the state is a camper's paradise, whether you've come to fish, paddle, swim, or hike. Thousands of miles of trails await backpackers and mountain bikers—plus you have the North Country Trail winding its way along the length of both peninsulas.

Water tends to be the real attraction here, and it is water that has largely determined Michigan's history. When major transportation routes were synonymous with rivers and lakes, the Great Lakes constituted a great highway. European explorers found they could penetrate deeper into the continent without the grueling job of hauling supplies and gear through untamed forest and over unfamiliar mountains if they simply loaded a canoe and followed the water. Of course, hauling a boat and luggage over rapids and across miles of portage was no easy task, but it beat the alternatives.

With the advent of the locomotive and then the automobile, land routes began to dominate, and the great bodies of water that would continue to play an important role in transporting Michigan lumber, copper, and iron became an obstacle to the general east-to-west flow of the nation. If you look at a map today, none of the east–west cross-country interstates even cross into Michigan. Aside from I-75, which begins at the southern end of Florida and ends in Sault Ste. Marie, you won't find any interstates north of the southernmost third of Michigan's Lower Peninsula. Of course, cities don't base their value on their proximity to a freeway, but these transportation hubs can tell you a lot about where businesses and people are in the state.

All of this is an incredible gift to people who like to go camping in tents. While most of the state's industry is found in a small swath of southern counties, this leaves the rest of the state open. And while you'll find excellent places to camp in the southern Lower Peninsula, it is the northern part of the "mitten" and the Upper Peninsula where you find sprawling state and national forests with hundreds of excellent campgrounds.

Though I am a Michigan native, I have lived and traveled extensively through New England and the mountains and plains of Colorado. Returning to Michigan after grad school was a real treat, and I've taken great pleasure in introducing my wife (a native of Colorado) and now our children to camping in this great state.

People have their own reasons for getting out into nature: exercise, relaxation, the pride of self-sufficiency. Lately, people have begun to enjoy "technology fasts"—simply leaving the world of cell phones, e-mail, tweets, and Facebook status updates behind to reset the mind, to reestablish a natural rhythm to their thinking. Whatever your reasons, I hope you find this guide a helpful resource. Be sure to let me know what you think, and keep camping!

INTRODUCTION

● ●

A Word about This Book and Michigan Tent Camping

As I travel throughout Michigan, I always like to check out the local real estate listings—especially the magazines that feature vacation property. Even when home prices bottom out around the country, small vacation homes still list for hundreds of thousands of dollars—millions for homes on waterfront property. A 100-foot-wide lot on Lake Michigan can start at half a million dollars, just for the acreage.

Thousands of people carry a humbler dream of a cottage in the woods on one of Michigan's smaller inland lakes. And even those who can scrimp and save for a summer getaway are often disappointed when the lot next door is bought by a well-to-do family from the city who erects a gaudy McMansion 5 feet off the property line. It's a common story to hear of once-remote hideaways that now look like the very subdivisions their owners were trying to escape in the first place.

Thankfully, there is another way to enjoy the natural beauty of Michigan. In my mind, the best places to spend your free time are those graciously provided by the state-park system and the National Park Service, as well as by numerous counties and townships: Michigan's campgrounds. The choicest pieces of land around the state of Michigan have been set aside for the enjoyment of anyone with a tent and a few bucks. Million-dollar views can be had for less than the price of a cheap hotel—often for much less. Those willing to tackle a little adventure will enjoy remote beaches, waterfalls, and scenic woodland hikes far from the madding crowd.

The nearly 20 state parks along Lake Michigan, for example, boast miles of sandy beach (much of it rarely visited by more than a few visitors), wooded campsites, rivers and lakes for fishing, and an extensive collection of trails for hiking and biking. At Sleeping Bear National Lakeshore, campers can enjoy a secluded campsite, take a long walk on the beach, explore the dunes, and tour quaint towns and villages along US 31—maybe even make the scenic drive to Traverse City, northern Michigan's premier vacation city.

Michigan's Upper Peninsula, on the other hand, has some of the best wilderness camping in the Midwest at Isle Royale National Park and the Porcupine Mountains Wilderness State Park. The North Country Trail, which crosses seven states on its way from New York to North Dakota, follows the shore of Lake Superior, connecting the Porkies in the west with the Pictured Rocks National Lakeshore farther east. In the southwest Upper Peninsula, the Sylvania Wilderness Area has backcountry camping for those who carry their gear in a canoe rather than a backpack or car trunk.

Even close to Metro Detroit, state parks and southeast Michigan's Metroparks have stellar camp facilities close to town but worlds away from the strip malls and shopping centers of civilization.

I've camped all over Michigan, and in this guide I bring to you what I believe are the 50 finest campgrounds in the state for tent camping. Tent campers have a unique perspective when it comes to spending their free time. More important to these folks than electricity, cable television, a game room, and level cement slabs is a picturesque wooded site that offers enough quiet and solitude to enjoy nature and the company of friends and family. My intention in writing this guide is to provide the information you need to make your next Michigan camping trip the best yet. I hope you enjoy these campgrounds as much as I have.

:: HARD CHOICES–ISLE ROYALE NATIONAL PARK

Trying to whittle the list of 1,200 or so campgrounds in Michigan down to 50 is a daunting task. You may skim the sites here and find that your favorite didn't make the cut. I'll be straight—a lot of great campgrounds didn't make the cut. Paddlers, anglers, mountain bikers, and hikers all have different requirements and preferences when it comes to camping. For aesthetic reasons, some folks enjoy a wide-open, grassy site overlooking a lake; others prefer a dark niche carved out of thick woods, set apart from the nearby river. I hope there's something in here for everyone.

That said, there is a notable omission here that needs special mention. While Michigan has the Sleeping Bear and the Pictured Rocks National Lakeshores, Isle Royale is technically the state's only national park. More than 40 miles north of the Keweenaw Peninsula in Lake Superior, Isle Royale National Park is composed of a long 207-square-mile island and the nearly 400 smaller islands that surround it.

To say the opportunities for camping at Isle Royale are numerous would be an understatement. (As this book focuses primarily on campgrounds, it seemed a shame to have to pick just one from the bunch and reduce the entire park to that description.) Backpacking routes traverse the island, from end to end. Ferries can get you to several campgrounds near the shore (though most visitors come to hike). Many people bring canoes and crisscross along the island's inland lake. Still others use sea kayaks to explore the island from the waters of Lake Superior. However you choose to enjoy the park, you share the wilderness with its full-time residents, including a thriving population of wolves and moose.

You will also find evidence of human history there—surprising in a place so remote. Native Americans were mining copper on the island as early as the fourth century B.C. These ancient mining sites are still visible, as are other pieces of the island's history, including lighthouses and shipwrecks.

Getting there is always the big question. Campers ferry to the island from Houghton, Michigan (a 6.5-hour trip); Copper Harbor, Michigan (a 4.5-hour trip); and Grand Portage, Minnesota (a 2- to 3-hour trip, depending on the ferry). This adds significantly to any trip. For example, if you live in or around Metro Detroit, the drive to Houghton is 9.5 hours. Once there, you find a room for the night and then wake the next morning to catch the ferry, another 6.5 hours to the first stop on the island. If your plans take you around to a campground on the island's far side, you could be looking at another day on the boat before you pitch your tent. That's two very full days before you even step onto Isle Royale.

The simple reason for omitting Isle Royale from this volume is that the park offers so much, and requires so much (in the way of skills, knowledge, and experience), that it really deserves an entire book to itself, and any mention we might make would be inadequate in preparing a camper for the experience. Fortunately, there is a book that offers the information you need to plan a trip of this scale. *Isle Royale National Park: Foot Trails & Water Routes* by Jim Dufresne is the guide to the island and has been used by thousands.

How to Use This Guidebook

:: THE RATINGS & RATING CATEGORIES

Evaluating campgrounds requires some finesse, and in the end it is more of an art than a science. For a quick summary of what qualities make these campgrounds worth visiting, each is rated on six attributes—beauty, privacy, spaciousness, quiet, security, and cleanliness. A five-star scale is used. Not every campground in this book can pull a high score in every category. Sometimes a very worthwhile campground is located on terrain that makes it difficult to provide a lot of space, for example. In these cases, look for high marks in beauty or quiet to trump room to stretch out. In every case, the star-rating system is a handy tool to help you pinpoint the campground that will fit your personal requirements.

★ ★ ★ ★ ★   The site is **ideal** in that category.
★ ★ ★ ★   The site is **exemplary** in that category.
★ ★ ★   The site is **very good** in that category.
★ ★   The site is **above average** in that category.
★   The site is **acceptable** in that category.

Beauty

Some campsites are so perfectly placed—nestled in cedars and white paper birch or on a bluff overlooking dunes—that it's hard to leave camp. Others are located with easy access to long stretches of Great Lakes shoreline with warm beaches and stunning sunsets (or sunrises, as the case may be). This rating accounts for both the beauty of the site and that of the general area.

Privacy

No one likes to duck out of a tent first thing in the morning to see neighbors brushing their teeth and spitting into the bushes just feet away. The best campgrounds keep sight lines to a minimum and allow bushes and trees to act as natural barriers.

Spaciousness

Fire pits quickly become a gathering place when folks are out camping. Campsites should have enough room for people to enjoy the fire with space to park the car, pitch a tent, and set up a dining area away from the flames. And if there's room for a hammock or clothesline, all the better.

Quiet

Some parks tend to attract a rowdy crowd from Memorial Day through Labor Day. Groups of children running through the campsites and grown-ups playing music long into the night are not everyone's idea of camping. Other campgrounds are relatively peaceful throughout the season. (Keep in mind, however, that any public campground can attract a party crowd, especially on holiday weekends. Thankfully, this situation isn't as likely at the more remote locations.)

Security

Campground hosts, park rangers, and gates that are closed after-hours can make a campground much more secure. Other campgrounds are far from civilization, and their remoteness can be both a source of security and a liability. In general, Michigan campgrounds are very safe, secure, and family-friendly.

Cleanliness

Each campground is rated on its overall cleanliness. Bathrooms and showers, camp stores, and other common areas are inspected and rated. It is also important that the sites themselves are clear of litter and the reminders of previous campers.

:: THE CAMPGROUND PROFILE

The campground profile is where you will find the nitty-gritty details. Not only is the property described, but readers can also get a general idea of the recreational opportunities available— what's in the area and perhaps suggestions for touristy activities.

:: THE OVERVIEW MAP, MAP KEY, AND LEGEND

To find the best campground in a specific part of the state, begin with the overview map (on the inside front cover of the book). The map shows you where all 50 campgrounds are located. The numbers in the diamonds correspond with the campgrounds on the facing page.

The book is organized by region, as indicated in the table of contents. A map legend that details the symbols found on the campground layout maps appears on the inside back cover.

:: CAMPGROUND-LAYOUT MAPS

Each chapter includes a small map. Campsites are shown, as well as the available facilities. Note that, in recent years, budget cuts have required the state to reduce the size of some campgrounds (and to close others). These maps are as accurate as we could make them, but conditions on the ground can change.

:: GPS CAMPGROUND-ENTRANCE COORDINATES

Backpackers and campers were the first group to adopt GPS technology. Now it seems everyone has a box squawking directions on their dashboard. As GPS tools have become more affordable, it makes sense to include that information in each chapter. This book gives each campground's location in latitude–longitude format.

:: WEATHER

Michigan weather is rather predictable. Rain is pretty common in the spring and fall. Throughout the summer, temperatures are warm and the air can be very humid—thunderstorms are common. Though the weather faithfully follows the seasons, the seasons themselves are not consistent throughout the state. Summer in the Upper Peninsula begins much later and ends much sooner. Fall colors that blaze in the Upper Peninsula in September take a month or more to reach the lower half of the Lower Peninsula. Even in the height of summer, the nights up north can be chilly. Closer to the lakes, weather changes more rapidly, but weather stations often have a good idea of what's coming ahead of time.

Tornadoes are a concern during their traditional season, which begins in spring and stretches into summer (but be aware that tornadoes have been reported year-round). In the event of a tornado, seek shelter. If you are caught out in the open, lie down in any sort of ditch you can find.

:: ANIMAL AND PLANT HAZARDS

Michigan's wildlife rarely causes campers much difficulty. Deer, of course, are always a road hazard toward dusk—on average, the state witnesses 40,000 car–deer crashes annually. Most occur in the southern half of the Lower Peninsula, but that's probably because there is more traffic in that region of the state.

Ticks

Ticks are not as much of a problem in Michigan as they are in other states. The most common tick you will encounter is the small hard tick. These arthropods are typically found on low-hanging branches waiting for unsuspecting passersby (they're hoping for deer). Tick-borne illness is not unheard of, and Lyme disease and Rocky Mountain spotted fever are just two of the illnesses that ticks can carry. After a hike through wooded and heavily grassy areas, it's a good idea to have a partner take a look at your back to be sure none of these buggers have nestled in. If you do find one embedded in your skin, use fine-tipped tweezers to pinch the tick as near to the skin as possible, and slowly pull straight up. If you later feel ill, or if a red ring appears around the removal site, see a doctor.

Blackflies

In the Upper Peninsula especially, blackflies are prodigious enough to make any camper downright ornery. From mid-May to July, their populations swell; with their painful bite, they can make outdoor activity north of the bridge unbearable. Repellents are not terribly effective, and most die-hard outdoor enthusiasts who brave the fly season recommend long-sleeved shirts and pants and even nets to protect your head and neck.

Mosquitoes

Though some illnesses are carried by mosquitoes, in Michigan these insects are more a nuisance than anything else. Repellents powered by DEET have proved the most effective; if you don't like the chemical on your skin, wear long sleeves and pants and spray your clothing.

Black Bears

Most campers who get a look at one of Michigan's black bears are more excited at the opportunity than frightened. Fewer than 20,000 of these notoriously shy bears roam the northern woods—90% of those are in the Upper Peninsula. When camping in bear country, be sure to keep your camp clean. Properly dispose of garbage and store food in a vehicle or a hanging "bear bag." Black bears are shy and typically avoid humans. If approached by a bear, try to scare it off by yelling and making yourself look big. If a bear attacks, fight back, beating it off with any implement at hand. Playing dead is not an effective strategy with a black bear.

Poison Ivy

More common than a black bear but harder to come by than a mosquito, poison ivy can make a trip very uncomfortable—and for those who are allergic, it can be deadly. The plant is recognizable by its three leaves ("leaves of three, let it be"). The oil in the plant causes a painful, itchy rash when it comes in contact with the skin. If you discover you've crunched through a patch of poison ivy, vigorously wash your exposed skin as soon as possible. (My grandma taught us to use Lava soap to remove the oil before a rash springs up, and that has seemed to work for me in the past.) The oil from the plant can stay on your clothes for a long time if not washed—and it's not unheard of for someone to get a second inflammation a year later after picking up a pair of shoes that weren't properly cleaned.

:: FIRST-AID KIT

A first-aid kit is an essential piece of gear, especially if your camping trips involve hiking, mountain biking, or other recreational activities. However, even collecting wood for the evening fire has its share of risks. Outfitters, such as REI and Moosejaw, sell prepackaged kits, as do places such as Target and Walmart. Read the label and be sure the kit you purchase (or assemble) has the following:

- Ace bandages
- Butterfly bandages
- Adhesive bandages (e.g., Band-Aids)
- Gauze and compress pads
- Moleskin
- Aspirin or acetaminophen

- Antibiotic ointment (e.g., Neosporin)

- Hydrogen peroxide

- For mild allergies: antihistamine

- For serious allergies: epinephrine

- Matches (in a waterproof container) or lighter

- Tweezers (for removing ticks)

- Whistle

- Signaling mirror

- Emergency/survival blanket

New campers should consider taking a first-aid class or, at the very least, picking up one of the many "quick guides" to first aid that you can find at your favorite outfitter.

:: PLANNING THE PERFECT TRIP

The key to any successful camping trip is in the planning. As we Boy Scouts recited in mantralike fashion, "The prepared scout is a happy scout." For me, this has proven true more often than not. For car campers who keep a vehicle nearby, there is no good reason not to bring along those little extras—an extra pair of socks, an extra wool blanket, and such.

- **Reserve Your Campsite**   Camping is popular in Michigan, and certain campgrounds are completely booked even before the season is underway. Last-minute campers will almost always find a site somewhere, but those who want a particular "somewhere" will need to plan ahead. Michigan state parks and recreation areas use the website **midnrreservations.com** for online reservations at all of their campgrounds. Sites at the national parks can be reserved through **recreation.gov**. Other campgrounds can be called in advance.

- **Prepare for the Weather**   It goes without saying that raingear is essential. Campers also need warm clothing, especially in the spring and fall. When consulting the weather forecast before a trip, be sure to note the nighttime lows. Many campers who come prepared only for 60-degree days will spend an awful night shivering when it drops into the 30s. Other essentials include a pack of playing cards and a book or two. If you have to be stuck in a tent all day, better have something to do.

- **Consider Your Tent Site**   The best place to pitch your tent is on level ground. Avoid tree roots and rocks. Also try to imagine where water might flow if it rains. Often the smoothest ground is that which has been washed clean by regular runoff from a nearby hill. And to avoid mosquitoes infiltrating your temporary abode, try to keep some distance from bushes and tall grass.

■ **Consider Your Camping Colleagues**   One of Ernest Hemingway's characters famously said, "Never go on trips with anyone you do not love." The question I would ask is, "How do you know you love someone until you've gone on a trip together?" A camping trip can be a great bonding experience. But realize that everyone approaches the art of camping from a different perspective. You need to make allowances when camping with new people. I once sat waiting for dinner while two friends argued over the amount of time it takes to boil water before it's safe to drink. One said 3 minutes; the other said 10. (Interestingly, if you search online for this information, you will find the same debate still raging among supposed experts.) After a few days, this kind of argument can ruin a trip. It's always best to remain gracious in the woods.

:: CAMPING ETIQUETTE

■ **Be a Good Neighbor**   The Golden Rule, "Treat your neighbor as you your-self would like to be treated," applies to camping as much as it does to life in general. Watch your noise in camp. Don't leave your garbage about. And keep the kids from running willy-nilly through others' sites.

■ **Follow the Rules**   You've heard that good fences make good neighbors? Campground rules are established to maintain a sense of order in a public place used by many different people. Not only do the rules help campground staff go about their business, they act as a fence between campers. In general, things like following the posted quiet hours and taking care of your trash help to maintain amiable relations between strangers.

■ **Respect the Wilderness**   When camping in wilderness areas, follow a strict carry in-carry out policy. It's frustrating when others leave a mess behind, thereby spoiling the experience for those who follow.

■ **Buy the Proper Permits**   The biggest change since the first edition of the book has been the creation of the Michigan Recreation Passport, which is purchased by residents when they register their automobile plates. The old sticker system is no longer around, and campers now need that little p on their tags to camp at state park and state forest campgrounds. Out-of-state visitors will want to stop at a state park and secure the necessary permits before they head out to a state forest campground. Some national parks also require a vehicle permit in addition to the camping fee. Though you may feel like you're getting nickel-and-dimed to death, these fees provide the neces-sary funds to pay park staff and maintain the campgrounds we love.

:: CANOE CAMPING

Michigan isn't Minnesota, where the canoe is practically ingrained into the camping culture, but the states do share many traits, and wilderness paddlers have plenty of waterways to keep them occupied. Rivers, lakes, ponds, and streams are everywhere. In Michigan, you are never more than 6 miles from an inland lake. As such, the region is especially suited for wilderness paddling. Even in southeast Michigan, within minutes of the 'burbs, state recreation areas have special campsites set aside for paddlers.

:: ROASTING MARSHMALLOWS

An important topic that often goes ignored in camping guides is a proper discussion of marshmallows. The name of this delicious treat comes from the *Althaea officinalis,* or common marshmallow, a flowering plant whose leaves, flowers, and roots were used for their medicinal properties. The ancient Egyptians were perhaps the first to see the confectionary value of the marshmallow, but it wasn't until the French added egg white and rose water to create pâté de guimauve that we saw a treat resembling the marshmallows we buy today. Interestingly enough, commercially available marshmallows these days are made primarily of sugar with some other ingredients to fluff them up (that is, "no marshmallows were harmed in the making of these marshmallows").

No one knows, of course, who came up with the idea of toasting marshmallows over an open fire. Whoever it was deserves a statue somewhere. Seriously. More than a tasty treat, roasted marshmallows have become a time-honored tradition here in the United States. When friends get together to sit around a campfire, it's time to gather some long sticks or roasting forks and open a bag of marshmallows. This warm, sugary treat is even better when stuffed between two graham crackers with a square of chocolate.

A certain etiquette applies when it comes to roasting marshmallows over a campfire. Most of the rules are just different ways of respecting individual preferences, because people come at the task different ways. Some are attracted to the flicker of the flame and delight as sugar is transformed into heat, what we call the flaming torch–mallow. Then there are the contemplative types, campers who carefully lay claim to the white-hot heat of the coals and slowly turn their sticks to create that perfect allover tan.

Whatever your inclination—whether you like your marshmallows hard in the middle with a crunchy black shell or lightly toasted yet warmed through and through (personally, I like a golden trunk topped with a slightly charred mushroom cap of burnt sugar)—as my daughter's Berenstain Bears video teaches, "People like different things, and that's okay."

For practical purposes, having enough sticks on hand is as important as remembering the Hershey's bars. When you only have one stick, the roaster is commonly expected to wait until everyone's had a bite before joining in. This can be a rough wait.

When there are enough roasting sticks for the whole gang, it's important to respect boundaries. That is, don't cross sticks. When someone is carefully rotating a marshmallow for the perfect golden color, reaching over his stick with your stick can prevent the timely removal of the marshmallow from the heat. Pretty soon, someone's not paying attention, sticks clash, and everyone's marshmallows end up in the ashes.

It's also wise, with so many people leaning over an open fire with hot melted sugar on the end of pointy sticks or metal roasting forks, to pay attention. Marshmallows on the ground can be a bummer, but it's only fun and games until someone gets a poker in the eye.

Southeast Michigan

1

Port Crescent State Park Campground

This quiet campground sits adjacent to 3 miles of sandy Lake Huron beach.

If you picture the flow of tourists surging north during the summer months as a river, the Thumb region of Michigan is a quiet eddy, off by itself. Bypassed by major highways, this part of the state has its own rhythms as the current takes the great mass of warm-weather travelers north and west, to Lake Michigan, to Grand Traverse Bay, to Mackinac. In a way, this makes no sense. The Thumb is surrounded by Lake Huron (the second largest of the Great Lakes), and the Saginaw Bay offers warm, shallow water; sandbars that go out forever; and miles of beautiful beaches—all just an hour or so from the state's largest urban center.

What might be disappointing for a struggling business in Port Austin,

however, is great news for campers. Two state parks sit on Lake Huron near the tip of the Thumb: Albert E. Sleeper and Port Crescent. With more than 200 sites, Albert Sleeper is the larger of the two, and it's not a bad place for camping. It sits back from the water, on the other side of the highway, in fact, and campers access the park beach by way of a pedestrian bridge. The Port Crescent campground, however, has almost half the number of campsites as its neighbor and is tucked in along the water. While the former has a fine reputation with campers, many of whom return year after year, I've developed a preference for the latter.

The park straddles the Pinnebog River. The day-use area, west of the river, has plenty of parking for beachgoers. There's a fitness trail and a fun day-use hiking trail. East of the river, next to the Old Pinnebog River Channel, is the campground. All told, the state park has 640 acres on Lake Huron.

The campground loop, with its 137 sites, is laid out lengthwise, so there are plenty of spaces to pitch a tent. The sites

:: Ratings

BEAUTY: ★ ★ ★ ★ ★
PRIVACY: ★ ★ ★
SPACIOUSNESS: ★ ★ ★ ★ ★
QUIET: ★ ★ ★ ★
SECURITY: ★ ★ ★ ★ ★
CLEANLINESS: ★ ★ ★ ★ ★

:: Key Information

ADDRESS: 1775 Port Austin Road, Port Austin, MI 48467

OPERATED BY: Michigan DNR-Port Crescent State Park

CONTACT: 989-738-8663; michigan.gov/portcrescent

OPEN: April-November

SITES: 137

EACH SITE: Picnic table and fire pit

ASSIGNMENT: Reservations can be made online at midnrreservations.com or by calling 800-447-2757.

REGISTRATION: Register at park office.

FACILITIES: Electricity, water, hot showers, modern restrooms, and pit toilets

PARKING: At site only

FEE: $27

ELEVATION: 590 feet

RESTRICTIONS:

■ **Pets:** On leash only

■ **Fires:** Fire pits only

■ **Alcohol:** Permitted

■ **Vehicles:** Michigan Recreation Passport required

■ **Other:** 15-day stay limit

along the water, however, are the best of the lot. The campground is, of course, very sandy, but campsites are tucked into the woods that skirt the beach. The view from the campground faces the northwest. Because the earth executes its annual tilt every summer, the sun's arc shifts northward, and the region's late evening sunsets are perfectly spotted for campers on the inside shore of the Thumb.

The park sits on the former site of Port Crescent, a boom town that cashed in on the region's lumber. It's hard to imagine now, but there was once a schoolhouse and a church here, as well as a hotel and a tavern. Sawmills lined the Pinnebog River, processing logs floating out from the interior. All that's left today is a bridge and the chimney monument, once part of a large brick sawmill.

The lumber boom that gave birth to the village of Port Crescent played an important role in the history of the region. Few people today remember the Fire of 1871, which destroyed millions of acres in Michigan. That story has been overshadowed by two other fires that started at the same time—the Peshtigo Fire in Wisconsin and the Chicago Fire (for which Mrs. O'Leary's unfortunate cow was to be the scapegoat). The Fire of 1871 would be the most destructive conflagration in Michigan history, but for the Thumb region it was just a dry run for the Great Thumb Fire of 1881.

In the intervening years, a wave of settlers moved in and put down roots here. So on September 5, 1881, when hurricane-force winds and high heat pushed a ravenous fire across the Thumb, it not only

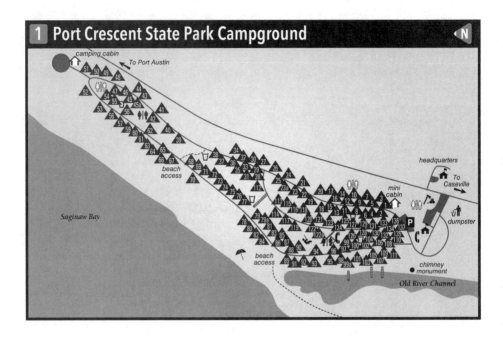

1 Port Crescent State Park Campground

camping cabin
To Port Austin
headquarters
To Caseville
mini cabin
beach access
dumpster
Saginaw Bay
beach access
chimney monument
Old River Channel

devoured more than a million acres, but it also killed 282 people and left thousands homeless. In a way, however, these fires helped clear the land for tenacious settlers who continued to come to farm.

Today, the Thumb region of the state depends on its agriculture. Farmers grow navy beans and sugar beets. The Michigan Sugar Company takes these beets and produces the Pioneer and Big Chief brands of sugar. But along the coast,

tourism remains a persistent, if not quiet, industry. The arc of M 25 connects the tourist towns of Port Huron, Lexington, Port Austin, Caseville, and Bay City. Port Crescent State Park is close to Port Austin and an easy drive from Caseville (and the ever-growing Cheeseburger in Caseville Festival). With sites close to the water and 3 miles of sandy beach, the park offers a quiet escape, right in the heart of things.

:: Getting There

M 25 makes a huge arc, tracing the Thumb from Bay City to Port Huron. From points west, take I-75 to Bay City (Exit 162) and follow M 25 east. From the Metro Detroit area, get on I-69 and head north on M 24 (for Lapeer, Exit 155) or M 53 (for Imlay City, Exit 168). The park is between those two roads on M 25.

GPS COORDINATES   N44° 0.414'   W83° 3.100'

2

Holly Recreation Area:
MCGINNIS LAKE CAMPGROUND

Just beyond the reach of the suburbs, Holly Rec offers many Michiganders the feel of Up North without the drive.

Located in northern Oakland County, the Holly Recreation Area is nearly 8,000 acres of steep rolling hills and small woodland lakes, the indelible reminders of the glaciers that once covered our humble peninsula. To put that into perspective, the acreage at Holly Rec adds up to 12.5 square miles. The state has turned the area into a showcase park for outdoor recreation. There is something here for everyone—miles of trails for hiking and cross-country skiing, beaches for swimming, and lakes for paddling and fishing. The park maintains one of the area's best disc golf courses. The course has 24 baskets, with routes that allow players to toss for 9, 18, or 24 holes.

Separate from the main park—west of the expressway on Grange Hall Road— Holly Rec also has trails set aside solely for mountain biking. These trails are serious business, with three loops (graded for ability) that add up to more than 23 miles of off-road pedaling.

The main day-use area and the campground are separated by McGinnis Road. If you are looking for a campground that's just a short walk away from the swimming beach, this isn't it. (For that, check out the Metamora-Hadley State Recreation Area.) It's at least a mile from the campground to the park's Heron Lake. However, what might be an inconvenience for some is a boon for others. You would be amazed at how many of the thousands who visit the park aren't even aware there is a campground here, which is surprising because it's not a small campground.

All told, there are 159 campsites, on five different loops, in the McGinnis Lake Campground. Of those, 144 are designated modern sites, meaning they have electrical service and modern restrooms. The remaining 15 semimodern sites (that

:: Ratings

BEAUTY: ★ ★ ★ ★
PRIVACY: ★ ★ ★
SPACIOUSNESS: ★ ★ ★ ★
QUIET: ★ ★ ★
SECURITY: ★ ★ ★ ★
CLEANLINESS: ★ ★ ★ ★ ★

:: Key Information

Address: 8100 Grange Hall Road, Holly, MI 48442

OPERATED BY: Michigan DNR–Holly State Recreation Area

CONTACT: 248-634-8811; **michigan.gov/holly**

OPEN: April–October

SITES: 15 semimodern; 144 modern

EACH SITE: Picnic table and fire pit

ASSIGNMENT: Reservations can be made online at **midnrreservations.com** or by calling 800-447-2757.

REGISTRATION: Register at park office.

FACILITIES: Electricity, water, hot showers, modern restrooms, and pit toilets

PARKING: At site only

FEE: $16 for semimodern sites; $23 or $21 for modern

ELEVATION: 1,028 feet

RESTRICTIONS:

■ **Pets:** On leash only

■ **Fires:** Fire pits only

■ **Alcohol:** Permitted, campground only

■ **Vehicles:** Michigan Recreation Passport required

■ **Other:** 14-day stay limit

is, sites without electricity) are all located on the Aspen Loop. These might seem like the best bet for tent campers. The loop, however, is wide open. The sites back up to some trees, but there are precious few trees between campsites, and that can make it feel like you're camping in a field. The modern sites, with their fancy electrical hookups and paved parking areas, are more expensive, but many of those are located on quieter loops, cushioned from neighbors by the surrounding forest. The Trillium and Oak loops offer a nice sense of privacy—and both are connected by short paths with the park's stunning 6.4-mile Holly-Wilderness Trail.

Because the park is so close to urban life, it's not uncommon for weekends to host a party crowd from time to time. The park is generally good about enforcing quiet hours, but be aware that it can be uncomfortable if you are cursed with inconsiderate neighbors. (Another reason to reserve a modern site.)

The campground, and the entire park, has the feeling of being remote—surprising considering one side of the park butts up against Dixie Highway. When you trace Dixie south on a map, ignoring the M 24 nonsense, you see that the road is an extension of Woodward Avenue. This was once the old Native American trail that connected the Detroit River with settlements on the Saginaw River. Back in 1831, French social observer Alexis de Tocqueville and his traveling companion wanted to explore the wilds of America. This brought them to Detroit, where they hired horses. In Pontiac they hired a guide. And with that, they headed into the uncivilized frontier.

Tocqueville describes the country

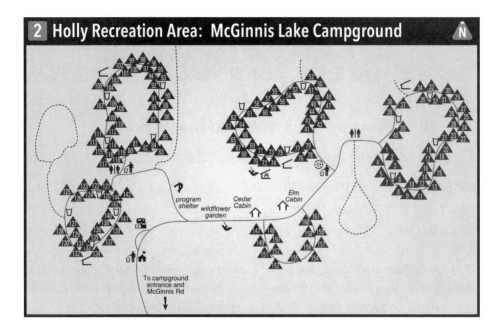

2 Holly Recreation Area: McGinnis Lake Campground

in his essay "Two Weeks in the Wilderness." He tells of small lakes "like a sheet of silver beneath the forest foliage," of a ground "intersected by hills and valleys," and of a "deep peace and an uninterrupted silence" (from Two Essays on America, translated by Gerald Bevan). Unfortunately, he also predicted that European settlers would eventually arrive, clearing the forest to make way for homesteads and farm fields. The best part of Holly Recreation Area—a bit of country Tocqueville surely passed on his way to Saginaw Bay—is that in some small way the park preserves that sense of deep peace and uninterrupted silence.

Of course, traffic can be heard dully humming in the background, and during the day the beach is packed with families playing in the water, but if you're looking to experience a bit of the primeval forest, a night at Holly Recreation Area is a good place to start.

:: Getting There

Near Clarkston, US 24 ends, but the road continues as Dixie Highway. Following Dixie Highway north, the park is southeast of the intersection with Grange Hall Road. From I-75–between Metro Detroit and Flint–take the Holly exit (Exit 101) for Grange Hall Road, and head east.

GPS COORDINATES   N42° 48.994'   W83° 31.515'

3

Pinckney Recreation Area:
CROOKED LAKE AND BLIND LAKE CAMPGROUNDS

You can pitch your tent on a wooded rise overlooking Blind Lake. In the evening, campers can relax to the sound of peepers in the nearby wetlands.

Northwest of Ann Arbor sits a rugged playground: the 11,000 acres of Pinckney Recreation Area. The park incorporates part of a larger terminal moraine area, which was formed at the end of a glacier—the soil is sandy and gravelly, the park is full of steep wooded hills, and the depressions in between them have become ponds and lakes. Taking full advantage of this unique terrain, the park has 26 miles of trails climbing in and around (and up and over) these hills. Pinckney Recreation Area and the neighboring Waterloo Recreation Area attract thousands of hikers and mountain bikers annually, and avid backpackers come for southern Michigan's longest hike, the

:: Ratings

BEAUTY: ★ ★ ★
PRIVACY: ★ ★ ★ ★
SPACIOUSNESS: ★ ★ ★ ★ ★
QUIET: ★ ★ ★ ★ ★
SECURITY: ★ ★ ★ ★
CLEANLINESS: ★ ★ ★ ★

36-mile Waterloo-Pinckney Trail, which was created to offer overnight hikers a multiday trip. The park is also popular with anglers who appreciate the dozens of small lakes and ponds.

In addition, the recreation area has three campgrounds. The one modern campground, Bruin Lake, with 186 sites, is the largest and most popular. Though relatively spacious and wooded, the sites are plotted like a parking lot, and this campground stays very busy all summer. It is not only visited by campers but also by folks looking to enjoy Bruin Lake for the day.

For a more secluded retreat, look for the 25 sites on Crooked Lake and the 10 sites on Blind Lake. The lack of warm showers and flush toilets keeps the less adventurous crowds away from these rustic campgrounds.

The sites on Blind Lake are found along the Potawatomi Trail, and campers have to either hike or bike into their camps. These sites are spaced with privacy in mind, and even the closest (2 and

:: Key Information

ADDRESS: 8555 Silver Hill Road, Pinckney, MI 48169

OPERATED BY: Michigan DNR–Pinckney Recreation Area

CONTACT: 734-426-4913; **michigan.gov/pinckney**

OPEN: May–October

SITES: 10 (Blind Lake); 25 (Crooked Lake)

EACH SITE: Picnic table and fire pit

ASSIGNMENT: Reservations can be made online at **midnrreservations.com** or by calling 800-447-2757.

REGISTRATION: Register (or self-register) at park headquarters.

FACILITIES: Water and vault toilets

PARKING: At site only; must park at Potawatomi Trailhead for Blind Lake sites

FEE: $12

ELEVATION: 922 feet

RESTRICTIONS:

- **Pets:** On leash only
- **Fires:** Fire pits only
- **Alcohol:** Permitted
- **Vehicles:** Michigan Recreation Passport required; no vehicles at Blind Lake
- **Other:** 15-day stay limit

3) have an obstructed sight line. Site 3 may be Pinckney's most desirable; you can pitch your tent on a wooded rise overlooking Blind Lake. In the evening campers can relax to the sound of peepers in the nearby wetlands.

The Potawatomi Trail makes a 17-mile loop through the eastern two-thirds of the park. Beginning at the parking lot in Silver Lake, it cuts a path west and north through dense woods, leg-burning hills, and sections of wheel-grabbing sand. Mountain bikers are supposed to ride clockwise, while hikers walk the loop counterclockwise. This way, hikers don't have to keep looking over their shoulders, and mountain bikers only have to worry about running into folks on foot around hidden corners.

On Saturday nights in the summer, this campground is often full. Reservations can be made online, or you can register at the park office before you hike in. Campers park at the day-use area and hike about 7 miles to the campground.

The 25 sites on the northeast shore of Crooked Lake are much more accessible. Many sites near the water have no trees for shade. Some sites have no natural dividing line and offer no privacy. There are, however, some real gems tucked in the woods away from the water. The campground has a boat launch and a fishing pier, which means anglers and boaters will keep the area busy on weekends. All told, choosing a site away from the water will greatly improve your stay. If water is a must, sites 21 and 22 are wooded and on the lake.

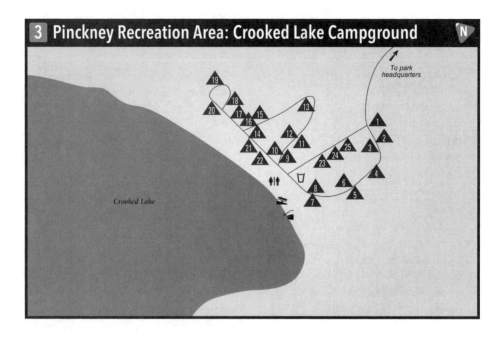

3 Pinckney Recreation Area: Crooked Lake Campground

Campers will find the best sites on the middle loop. Site 13 offers plenty of privacy, and sites 9 and 11 have room to spread out. I am also fond of sites 1–4. These are farthest from the water on grassy lots with shade.

The drive from the park office to the campground is 1.5 miles. When you register (or self-register after-hours) at the office, they ask that you first go out and pick a site. On a busy evening, campers have driven out to the campground, found a site, and returned to the office only to find that the site they selected was registered to another camper while they were out looking, someone they must have passed along the road. Register online ahead of time if you can. Otherwise, be prepared to leave a bag at your chosen site so that the next unfortunate camper doesn't come right behind you to register the same site.

Mountain bikers know Pinckney Recreation Area has some of the best trails in southeast Michigan—no rail-to-trail paved pathways here. This is New England–style singletrack. Rolling terrain, some tight technical areas, and a variety of loops keep it interesting. One unique feature is the sandy sections, which seem to pop up in the most unfortunate places (such as at the bottom of a hill, around a tight corner, or on a straightaway when you're looking for speed).

For hikers, the trails offer much more than a day of walking. The Waterloo-Pinckney Trail alone crosses 36 miles, connecting the park with the Waterloo Recreation Area. (This trail starts in Waterloo

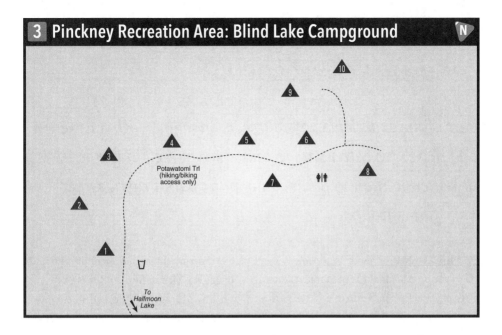

3 Pinckney Recreation Area: Blind Lake Campground

Potawatomi Trl
(hiking/biking
access only)

To
Halfmoon
Lake

for hikers walking west to east. See profile for Green Lake Campground, on page 22, for more information.) Hikers looking for a shorter walk in the woods can tackle the 5-mile loop out and around Crooked Lake or the 2-mile Silver Lake Trail. There are others as well, all accessed from the parking area on Silver Lake.

Silver Lake also offers better swimming than campers will find at Crooked Lake. And for folks who appreciate the amenities of a modern campground, there are flush toilets at Silver Lake, and campers can always drive over to the Bruin Lake Campground for a hot shower.

:: Getting There

The starting point for adventure at Pinckney begins on Silver Hill Road. From Dexter, take Dexter-Pinckney Road to North Territorial Road. Take that west to Dexter Town-hall Road north. The park entrance is 1 mile up on the west side of the road. From US 23, take the North Territorial Road (Exit 49) 10 miles west to Dexter Townhall Road. Turn north. The park is a mile up on the left.

GPS COORDINATES   N42° 25.308'   W83° 58.752'

4

Waterloo Recreation Area:
GREEN LAKE CAMPGROUND

Part of the experience, of course, is engaging with nature, and there's no better way to immerse yourself in the heart of Waterloo than to pitch camp in the park's rustic Green Lake Campground.

The **20,000** acres of Waterloo Recreation Area make it the largest state park in the Lower Peninsula. The park features the Gerald E. Eddy Discovery Center, where people come to learn about the local ecology, and the Waterloo Farm Museum, which is operated by the Waterloo Area Historical Society. Though the park shares many traits with the neighboring Pinckney Recreation Area—it has two modern campgrounds (to Pinckney's one), a swimming beach, and trails for hiking, biking, and horseback riding— Waterloo places more of an emphasis on interpreting the region's natural and human history for visitors.

:: Ratings

BEAUTY: ★ ★ ★ ★
PRIVACY: ★ ★ ★
SPACIOUSNESS: ★ ★ ★ ★ ★
QUIET: ★ ★ ★ ★ ★
SECURITY: ★ ★ ★ ★
CLEANLINESS: ★ ★ ★ ★ ★

Part of the experience, of course, is engaging with nature, and there's no better way to immerse yourself in the heart of Waterloo than to pitch camp in the park's rustic Green Lake Campground, which consists of 25 sites on a small loop. Sites overlook the lake on one side and back up to wetlands on the other. Encircling a small grassy knoll, many of the sites on the inside are out in the open, exposed both to the elements and to the eyes of nearby campers. Sites on the outside of the loop, however, are nestled in the trees and offer a little more privacy.

Site 8 offers the most privacy. Surrounded by trees, right on the water, the site is downhill from the main road that runs through the campground. Sites 5 and 6 also sit on the water. The wide, grassy lots have nice overhead coverage from the sun but little privacy. Sites 2 and 4, which sit across from these, also enjoy plenty of shade, but when someone decides to crank open a pop-up between

:: Key Information

ADDRESS: 16345 McClure Road, Chelsea, MI 48118

OPERATED BY: Michigan DNR–Waterloo Recreation Area

CONTACT: 734-475-8307; **michigan.gov/waterloo**

OPEN: March–December

SITES: 25

EACH SITE: Picnic table and fire pit

ASSIGNMENT: Reservations can be made online at **midnrreservations.com** and by calling 800-447-2757.

REGISTRATION: Self-register at campground.

FACILITIES: Water and vault toilets

PARKING: At site only

FEE: $12

ELEVATION: 965 feet

RESTRICTIONS:

- **Pets:** On leash only
- **Fires:** Fire pits only
- **Alcohol:** Permitted
- **Vehicles:** Michigan Recreation Passport required
- **Other:** 15-day stay limit

you and the water, it will most certainly block the view of the lake.

Waterloo boasts a 5-mile mountain-bike loop, but trail planners overlapped the trail with a longer bridle path, and in the past this has made the track unridable. Your best bet is to take your mountain bike next door. The miles of maintained singletrack at Pinckney will not disappoint.

Campers looking for a nice hike in the woods, or through a meadow or around a lake, are in for better luck. A network of nature hikes—14 miles of trails divvied up into seven loops ranging from 0.8 to 5.3 miles—all lead out from the Discovery Center. The Discovery Center draws thousands of visitors every year, including busloads of students. Run as a joint project by the Michigan Department of

Natural Resources and the Waterloo Natural History Association, the center sheds light on the region's unique geology and ecology. With its hands-on exhibits and displays and a full complement of programs for kids and families, you'll come away with a head full of knowledge about local birds and their plumage; the hive building of bees; ice ages, glaciers, and mammoths; Waterloo's trees and flowers; and even a little astronomy.

Among the area's geological peculiarities are its kettle lakes and bogs, part of the glacial influence on southeast Michigan. The bogs here are home to some of the most exotic plants in the state, in particular carnivorous pitcher plants and sundews, as well as wild irises. You might spot some of these when hiking the Bog Trail. Much of this path is on an elevated wooden walkway—no need to worry about returning with wet shoes.

Hikers looking for more than an afternoon stroll, however, will want to take note of the 36-mile Waterloo-Pinckney Trail, which connects the Pinckney Recreation Area (to the east, between Pinckney and Dexter) with the Waterloo Recreation Area (to the west, between Waterloo and Chelsea). The trail was designed to offer backpackers a multiday hike in southeast Michigan. Backpackers typically follow the trail west to east, beginning the trek at the modern Portage Lake campground. A day of hiking brings them to the park's other modern campground at Sugarloaf Lake. Ten miles farther, just before entering the Pinckney portion of the trail, hikers will often spend the night at the Green Lake Campground.

The portion of the trail that passes through the Waterloo Recreation Area is quite stunning, and I would recommend taking some time to hike a piece. Along the way, the path passes through woods and marsh as well as fields, which in the summer are covered with wildflowers. It climbs some interesting terrain and comes close to nearly a dozen lakes and ponds. The trail can be especially arresting in the fall, when the foliage begins to change color.

For an appreciation of what it must have been like to come to this area as a settler, head over to the Waterloo Farm Museum. In 1844, Johannes and Fredericka Ruehle moved their children into a log house here, and the museum tells the story of this family and their progeny. For more than a hundred years, the Realy family—Realy is the Americanized spelling of Ruehle—farmed this land, and their story sheds light on what life was like for many families across Michigan. From the farmhouse to the bakehouse and plenty of other structures in between, this is a great place to spend a few hours.

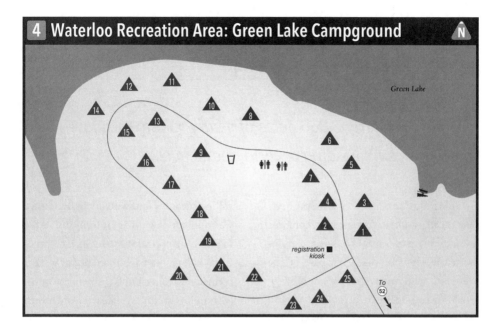

:: Getting There

The campground is on the eastern edge of the park. The entrance is off M 52, 5.5 miles north of I-94 (Exit 159).

GPS COORDINATES   N42° 21.846'   W84° 04.218'

5

Lake Hudson
Recreation Area

The park is nearly 2,800 acres of gently rolling meadow and woods surrounding a warm inland lake.

Lake Hudson is the most southerly campground in this book. In Lenawee County, the park entrance is just 9 miles from the Ohio border. This part of the state fits with many people's notion of the Midwest—miles of farmland and long drives broken up by small towns that the interstates have largely bypassed. And while northern Ohio and southern Michigan do not have the endless cornfield vistas of Iowa or Nebraska, the miles of open acreage broken up by distant hedgerows of trees and the occasional creek are just as uneventful to the uninitiated.

Many destinations (at least, here in the Great Lake State) dispel this stereotype, but Lake Hudson is in the heart of it. The park is nearly 2,800 acres of gently

:: Ratings

BEAUTY: ★ ★ ★ ★
PRIVACY: ★ ★ ★
SPACIOUSNESS: ★ ★ ★ ★ ★
QUIET: ★ ★ ★ ★
SECURITY: ★ ★ ★ ★
CLEANLINESS: ★ ★ ★ ★ ★

rolling meadow and woods surrounding a warm inland lake. It is far from the state's main transportation arteries—8 miles from US 127, a back-road highway that connects Lansing and Jackson to the north with points south. The nearest town with a significant population is Adrian, 15 miles to the east. Once you leave the highways, it's all country driving.

The campground is nearly 2 miles from the park entrance; the road passes through open meadow and areas forested with white birch, box elder, and mixed hardwoods. Along the way are turnoffs for the boat launch and the beach area. The campground is semimodern, meaning that most sites have electricity, but that's the extent of the modern amenities. The campground is divided into two sections—east and west—each with 25 campsites. Each section has a vault toilet, and they share a hand-pump well and a Dumpster.

There are few trees, and privacy was apparently not a factor when the sites were laid out. Thick brush does a great job of blocking the view of campers on

:: Key Information

ADDRESS: 5505 Morey Highway, Clayton, MI 49235

OPERATED BY: Michigan DNR–Lake Hudson Recreation Area

CONTACT: 517-445-2265; **michigan.gov/lakehudson**

OPEN: April–November

SITES: 50

EACH SITE: Picnic table and fire pit

ASSIGNMENT: Reservations can be made online at **midnrreservations.com** and by calling 800-447-2757.

REGISTRATION: Register at park office.

FACILITIES: Well water and vault toilets

PARKING: At site only

FEE: $16

ELEVATION: 865 feet

RESTRICTIONS:

■ **Pets:** On leash only

■ **Fires:** Fire pits or in waist-high stoves in the picnic area only

■ **Alcohol:** Permitted

■ **Vehicles:** Michigan Recreation Passport required

■ **Other:** 15-day stay limit

each side, but the view directly across is unobstructed. The campsites in the east section, specifically the even-numbered sites, back up to each other and offer the least in the way of privacy. Sites 10 and 14 are practically one open area. And sites such as 27 are so exposed that it's hard to imagine camping here without a trailer for privacy and an expansive awning for shade. For tent campers, many sites are open to the sun all day, which can make for an uncomfortable stay in the summer.

The west section has the choicest spots to pitch a tent. Sites 37 and 38 are wooded, more secluded, and right on the water. But even the sites here, away from the water, seem to offer more privacy.

The park's relatively flat geography and remote location make it a great spot for amateur astronomers. In 1993, the state legislature designated Lake Hudson as Michigan's first dark-sky preserve. (Michigan was the first state to set up a preserve like this on public land.) The lights of Detroit and Toledo are distant distractions on the horizon and are easily ignored when the Milky Way stretches across the night sky. Wherever lighting is necessary within the park, it is directed at the ground and shielded (operated with motion detectors, if possible).

It's not just astronomers who appreciate a dark night. As more and more of the planet is covered with artificial light, the night skies have grown noticeably dim, and not just in urban areas. City lights reflected off the atmosphere create a glare that obscures stars and other nighttime phenomena miles away. Just as many campers head to state parks and other campgrounds to escape the noise of civilization, so finding a dark-sky preserve such as this offers campers an opportunity to escape the visual noise of the city and suburbs as well.

Of course, overnight park visitors will need light. A late-night jog to the vault toilet without a flashlight is ill-advised, and the fire pits are not just for show. But visitors are asked to keep the use of lights at night to a minimum.

Day users come to the recreation area for Lake Hudson itself. The park has a decent beach, picnic area, and volleyball nets. The water gets warm in the summer and makes for great swimming. The day-use area is more than a mile away around a bend in the lake, and even on busy days it is out of sight for most campers. Spring, summer, and fall find anglers trolling the 600-acre lake, mainly looking to land muskies—the lake reputably has some of the largest around—but bluegill, largemouth and smallmouth bass, and walleye are not uncommon.

Gently rolling meadows, wetlands, and woods are perfect habitats for waterfowl, pheasants and turkeys, deer, and small game. Hunters make good use of the land in season.

July is the busiest camping season. May and the first half of June, as well as mid- to late August, are your best bets for finding one of the two or three really choice sites. Reservations can be made online or by calling 800-447-2757, but there's hardly a time you will find the campground completely full.

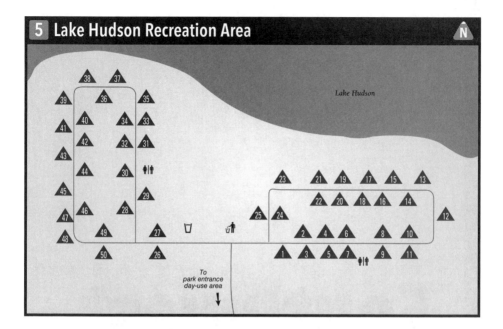

5 Lake Hudson Recreation Area

Lake Hudson

To
park entrance
day-use area

:: Getting There

From points west, take I-94 to US 127 south (Exit 142). Continue about 30 miles to M 34 (Main Street/West Carleton Road) east, in Hudson. Continue 6.5 miles to M 156 (Morey Highway) and head south a little more than a mile to the park entrance.

From the east, take US 23 south to Exit 5. Head west on US 223 for 20 miles. In Adrian, follow M 34 west for 12 miles, turning south on M 156 (Morey Highway). The park is about a mile south; you'll see the signs.

GPS COORDINATES   N41° 49.482'   W84° 15.576'

Southwest Michigan

6

Warren Dunes State Park:
RUSTIC CAMPGROUND

It's a nice campground with plenty of trails for hiking, dunes for climbing, and beaches for swimming.

The southwest corner of Michigan is the domain of Chicagoans. That may be overstating it a bit, but it's hard to understate the influence that Chicago has had on the development of tourism along this stretch of Lake Michigan shoreline. Dig a little into the history of many local restaurants and inns, and somewhere in their past you will likely find stories of some family from the Windy City who decided to move to southwest Michigan to make a go of it in the service industry. Of course, much of the coast has been built up on this side of the state, but folks from Illinois and Indiana, with just the weekend to recreate, find Harbor Country an easy drive.

:: Ratings

BEAUTY: ★ ★ ★ ★ ★
PRIVACY: ★ ★ ★ ★
SPACIOUSNESS: ★ ★ ★ ★ ★
QUIET: ★ ★ ★ ★ ★
SECURITY: ★ ★ ★ ★ ★
CLEANLINESS: ★ ★ ★ ★ ★

In the midst of marinas, public beaches, summer homes, and burger joints, Warren Dunes State Park offers a surprisingly pleasant natural retreat. That is not to say that the park stands as some bastion of solitude. With 3 miles of beach, a towering dune, and sand-side concessions and restrooms, the park can get downright crowded on sunny summer days. What often get overlooked are campgrounds. The park has two: one modern and one rustic.

Roads give visitors access only to the southern half of the park. The rustic campground lies along a loop at the northernmost end of the road. Campers can pitch their tents with the satisfaction of knowing that the milling crowds of sunbathers are more than 2 miles away in the day-use area. The rustic campground has 36 sites, which have fire pits and picnic tables and are serviced by four vault toilets and a well for water. Many of the sites, especially those along the eastern edge of the loop, are out in the open. Grassy and sunny, the ground is perfect for pitching a tent, though the sites offer

:: Key Information

ADDRESS: 12032 Red Arrow Highway, Sawyer, MI 49125

OPERATED BY: Michigan DNR–Warren Dunes State Park

CONTACT: 269-426-4013; **michigan.gov/warrendunes**

OPEN: April–October

SITES: 36

EACH SITE: Picnic table and fire pit

ASSIGNMENT: Reservations can be made online at **midnrreservations.com** and by calling 800-447-2757.

REGISTRATION: Register at park office.

FACILITIES: Well water and vault toilets

PARKING: At site

FEE: $16

ELEVATION: 651 feet

RESTRICTIONS:

- **Pets:** On leash only
- **Fires:** Fire pits only
- **Alcohol:** Prohibited April–September
- **Vehicles:** Michigan Recreation Passport required
- **Other:** 15-day stay limit

little privacy. Even those in the woods along the other side of the loop have little undergrowth to screen the neighbors.

The best site of the bunch has to be site 1 (and 2 is a close runner-up). Because the campground is on a one-way loop, all sites experience the same amount of traffic. Right at the entrance, however, bushes and trees offer campers a feeling of solitude. I also think sites 24 and 26 are pretty nice, tucked into the trees as they are.

The modern campground, on the other hand, is much larger. It has 184 sites on two large loops, each divided by an extra row of campsites. There are modern restrooms with hot showers, playgrounds for the kids, and even a small general store. Even with all the hoopla, this campground would make a fine alternative if the rustic sites were booked or if your party includes campers who prefer to be a little closer to flush toilets. The sites offer more privacy between neighbors, and the ground is a combination of packed earth and gravel and grass.

The attraction of the beach is obvious, but this strip of sand is a bare fraction of the park's 1,952 acres. If you were to walk inland from Lake Michigan, up and over the foredunes and the backdunes, your path would trace the life cycle of a dune, from the active modern dunes by the lake to ancient dunes covered in a climax forest of beech and maple. The dips in between the parallel rows of hills contain unique biological ecosystems. In spring and early summer, you will find swaths of wildflowers; in the fall, the maples turn to vibrant shades of orange and red.

Allowing visitors access to the more remote portions of the park, 6 miles of trails wind through Warren Dunes. You can find trailheads at the end of the beach parking lot and in both campgrounds. The dune environment, built on sand as it is, tends to be fragile; as such, the paths are designated for hiking and cross-country skiing—no horses and no mountain bikes.

The very existence of this natural preserve in the heart of Harbor Country is the result of one man's foresight. E. K. Warren, a businessman from Three Oaks, purchased the property in 1880. The land wasn't much use for farming, and locals considered the property so worthless that many allowed ownership to revert to the state in lieu of paying property tax. Needless to say, his purchase was considered foolish at best. In 1930, the dunes were established as a state park. (For another of Warren's preserves, check out the Warren Woods State Park, 3 miles north of Three Oaks.)

The park has not been immune to a series of blights that have destroyed trees in recent years. In response to the emerald ash borer beetle, more than 4,000 trees were removed from the park. It's easy to imagine what impact this has had on the landscape, though first-time visitors may not notice the loss.

Still, it's a nice campground with plenty of trails for hiking, dunes for climbing, and beaches for swimming. All this, and a cheeseburger at Redamak's Tavern in New Buffalo is just a 10-minute drive away.

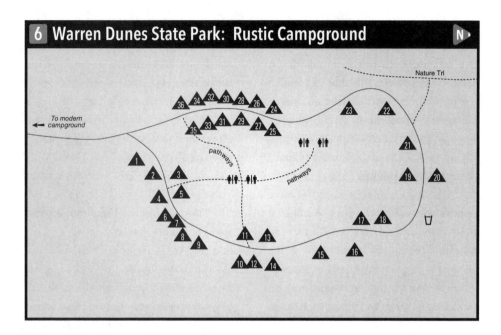

:: Getting There

At Exit 16 off I-94, take the Red Arrow Highway south. The park entrance is down a little more than 2 miles on the right.

GPS COORDINATES   N41° 54.636'   W86° 35.304'

7

Yankee Springs State Recreation Area:

DEEP LAKE RUSTIC CAMPGROUND

The trailhead for one of southwest Michigan's best mountain-biking rides is found near the entrance of the campground.

Rustic campgrounds in Michigan tend to be low-key. Typically, the state forest service will plot a couple dozen sites near a lake or river, dig a pit or two for vault toilets, drill a hole for a hand-pumped well, and throw up a sign welcoming campers to XYZ Campground. It's a formula that works and has come to define a level of roughing it that is replicated all over the state. If a campground grows much larger than this, you start finding flush toilets and hot showers, and then it's not long before someone is paving sites for RVs and closing sites to build comfy minicabins for the tentless.

Yankee Springs Recreation Area bucks this trend. In addition to a hugely popular

modern campground on Gun Lake, the park maintains what may be the largest rustic campground in the state. More than 3.5 miles away on the eastern edge of the park, Deep Lake Rustic Campground has 120 sites on four loops. Each loop is poised on the top of a bluff overlooking the water. The campground sits high, maybe 50 feet, above the lake, and no sites are along the shore; the drop is simply too steep. This unique configuration results in loops that are quite separate from each other. You may see the outline of a neighbor's tent through the woods, but between loops the land dips into small ravines.

The lower-numbered sites in the two northernmost loops tend to be paired together. Sites 17 and 18, for example, have their own picnic tables and fire pits, but they share the same clearing in the trees—offering virtually no privacy unless your party takes up both sites. Sites such as 38, 39, and 41 have a great view of the water, but none are right on it.

The two southernmost loops—sites 86–95 and 98–116—are smaller, more

:: Ratings

BEAUTY: ★ ★ ★ ★ ★
PRIVACY: ★ ★ ★
SPACIOUSNESS: ★ ★ ★ ★
QUIET: ★ ★ ★ ★
SECURITY: ★ ★ ★ ★ ★
CLEANLINESS: ★ ★ ★ ★ ★

:: Key Information

ADDRESS: 2104 South Briggs Road, Middleville, MI 49333

OPERATED BY: Michigan DNR–Yankee Springs State Recreation Area

CONTACT: 269-795-9081; michigan.gov/yankeesprings

OPEN: April–November

SITES: 120

EACH SITE: Picnic table and fire pit

ASSIGNMENT: Reservations can be made online at midnrreservations.com and by calling 800-447-2757.

REGISTRATION: Register at park office, or self-register if office is closed.

FACILITIES: Well water and pit toilets

PARKING: At site

FEE: $12

ELEVATION: 867 feet

RESTRICTIONS:
- **Pets:** On leash only
- **Fires:** Fire pits only
- **Alcohol:** Prohibited
- **Vehicles:** Michigan Recreation Passport required
- **Other:** 15-day stay limit

intimate, and deeper into the woods. In the distance, you can view the lake through the trees, but generally these sites are more private. On the side of the road, between clumps of campsites, sites 106 and 107 are particularly set apart—not on the water but with nice scenery nonetheless.

The trailhead for one of southwest Michigan's best mountain-biking rides is found near the entrance of the campground. Thirteen miles of trail, ranging from easy to technical, take riders throughout the northeast portion of the recreation area. Along the way, the path passes Devil's Soupbowl (a glacially carved kettle formation), Graves Hill Overlook (just what it sounds like), and The Pines (an area of tall trees planted in the 1940s).

A sign at the trailhead for the bike path reads TRAILS PASS THROUGH OPEN HUNTING AREAS: WEAR BRIGHT COLORS. Take notice. Hunting is popular here and in the neighboring Barry State Game Area. This is the kind of advice that, if neglected, will suddenly come to mind when you're a mile into the woods and hear not-so-distant gunshots.

On laid-back summer weekends, Yankee Springs attracts big crowds. Thankfully for tent campers, most steer clear of Deep Lake (which doesn't have a beach). Gun Lake is the prime destination for sunbathing and swimming. Along Murphy's Point, which juts out into the lake just south of the modern campground, the park maintains three sandy beaches and a boat launch. The point's three large parking areas, bathhouses, picnic areas, and concessions give beachgoers everything they need for a day on the water.

Anglers will find access for fishing on most of the lakes in Yankee Springs, and these are all easy to get to from Gun Lake Road or Chief Noonday Road.

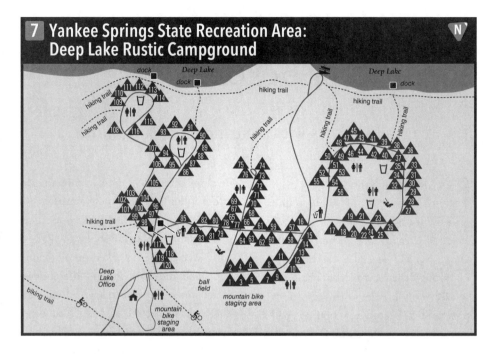

Those interested in Michigan's history —especially stories of its native peoples— will be interested to know about Chief Noonday (known alternatively as Nau-on-qual-que-zhick and Nau-qua-ga-sheek). In the early 19th century, he was chief of the Ottawa in a village that is now Grand Rapids. He later settled south of here in Prairieville, and the Yankee Springs area is known as a place where his people hunted game. History tells us that he fought on the side of the British in the War of 1812 and later signed treaties with the American government, surrendering huge tracts of Ottawa land, thus opening up Ohio and Michigan for settlement.

Chief Noonday's legacy lives on. Grand Rapids recently unveiled a statue to commemorate his life, and his name is tacked on to local streets and, in the park, a lake, trail, and nature center. If traditional accounts can be trusted, he lived to be nearly 100 years old and died here in Barry County.

:: Getting There

North of Kalamazoo, take US 131 to Exit 61. Drive east on 129th Avenue 7.5 miles to Briggs Road, and turn right. Four miles on (the road has turned into Gun Lake Road), you will come to South Yankee Springs Road. Turn left, and the park is a half mile up on the left (west) side of the road.

GPS COORDINATES   N42° 37.026'   W85° 27.192'

8

Highbank Lake National Forest Campground

The area verily bristles with recreational opportunities.

The **Manistee** National Forest maintains a handful of campgrounds between the towns of Baldwin and White Cloud, all close to M 37. The Pere Marquette River and several of its tributaries run through this part of the forest, and the area verily bristles with recreational opportunities—camping, hiking, paddling, and fishing, to name a few. Nearby, the North Country Trail winds around rivers and lakes, passing close enough to most of these campgrounds to be connected by short spurs.

Highbank Lake Campground is in good company. To the south, its neighbors are Benton Lake and Nichols Lake campgrounds; to the east, Shelley Lake; and, just a few miles north, Bowman Bridge (the only one of the lot on the Pere Marquette River). Though all are

:: Ratings

BEAUTY: ★ ★ ★ ★
PRIVACY: ★ ★ ★ ★
SPACIOUSNESS: ★ ★ ★
QUIET: ★ ★ ★ ★ ★
SECURITY: ★ ★ ★ ★ ★
CLEANLINESS: ★ ★ ★ ★

in close proximity, these campgrounds offer very different camping experiences. While the campground at Nichols Lake seems particularly convenient for RVs—with well-defined packed-gravel spurs and flush and vault toilets—the narrow rutted drive into the dispersed sites at Shelley Lake would be a tight squeeze for anything bigger than a humble SUV, and the campground doesn't even offer potable water or an outhouse. The campground at Highbank Lake strikes a balance between these two.

As the name suggests, the ground around the lake rises steeply from the water's edge. There's room enough for four campsites right on the lake, but the rest of the campground's nine sites are spotted on the rise, nestled under a canopy of oak and the occasional maple. Two in particular, sites 7 and 8, are a ways up the hill, requiring campers to park alongside the loop and hike up and in. With only nine sites and no way to make reservations, you take your chances camping here on peak summer weekends.

For tent camping, Highbank proves to be especially equipped. Only a few of these sites can accommodate RVs, and

:: Key Information

ADDRESS: 650 North Michigan Avenue, Baldwin, MI 49304

OPERATED BY: Huron-Manistee National Forest, Baldwin/White Cloud Ranger District

CONTACT: 231-745-4631; tinyurl.com/lmsexnu

OPEN: Mid-May–late September

SITES: 9

EACH SITE: Picnic table, fire pit with grill, and lantern post

ASSIGNMENT: First come, first served

REGISTRATION: Self-register at campground.

FACILITIES: Hand-pumped water and vault toilets

PARKING: At site

FEE: $16

ELEVATION: 885 feet

RESTRICTIONS:

■ **Pets:** On leash only

■ **Fires:** Fire pits only

■ **Vehicles:** 2 per site

campground facilities include a vault toilet and water from a hand-pump well. But the sloping terrain can present difficulties. Site 1, for example, offers campers great access to the water, but you have to watch the pitch when setting up your tent. It's easy to see how a sudden rainstorm could generate a mini deluge. Even in good weather, I imagine a poorly planned location would result in campers fighting the roll of gravity throughout the night. (None of these drawbacks, however, would keep me from trying to snag site 1 if it was available.)

In late summer, lying in your tent and listening to the sounds of the forest, you will hear the smack of acorns falling on the carpet of last year's leaves (and your tent, for that matter). Above the lake, ferns cover the forest floor on both sides of the drive in. If you miss the turn for the

campground, you will soon find yourself immersed in an intricate web of sandy doubletrack. Make a turn without paying special attention to landmarks, and you will drive around confused until you eventually emerge on some thoroughfare of substance. These Forest Service roads, however, would be nice for an evening walk or to explore with a mountain bike.

For more vigorous exploration of the Manistee National Forest, the North Country Trail (NCT) passes the western edge of Highbank Lake. The campground connects to the trail by way of a half-mile spur that follows the northern edge of the lake. You know you've found the trail when you see the blue-diamond blazes. Mountain bikes are prohibited on this stretch of the NCT, but cyclists will find access open to the trail north of the Bowman Lake Trailhead (near the Bowman Bridge

Campground) and south of Nichols Lake.

The NCT passes through, or close by, quite a few of the campgrounds listed in this book. That's no coincidence. When complete, the NCT will offer hikers an uninterrupted trail from the Adirondacks in New York to Lake Sakakawea in North Dakota, traversing seven states along the way—including the full lengths of both the Upper and Lower Peninsulas. To create a continuous trail on this scale, developers often work by connecting pre-existing paths. Trails that are connected to established networks (the kind with campgrounds) are especially necessary to building a successful thru-hike.

There's no formal boat launch here, just access enough to carry your canoe or small rowboat to the water. At only 20 acres, Highbank Lake might be a bit small for a weekend of cruising, but there are plenty of other lakes to explore by canoe and kayak, and the nearby Pere Marquette River is rightfully one of the state's premier paddling rivers.

Anglers at Highbank Lake pull in plenty of bluegill, panfish, and bass. Just southeast of Highbank Lake is the slightly larger Amaung Lake, which some suggest offers better fishing. It certainly offers more secluded fishing. Surrounded by national forest, with limited access by road (at best), Amaung defines "off the beaten path." According to national-forest maps, Forest Service Road 5561 (the first left on FS 5396 once you've turned off Roosevelt Road) will take you around to the northern end of the lake. However, if you simply walk south on 5396 (the one you came in on) for 500 yards past the campground entrance and then plunge southeast cross-country through the woods for several hundred feet, you're sure to stumble upon Amaung.

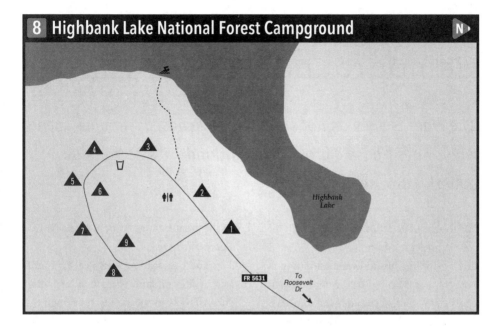

:: Getting There

Nine miles south of Baldwin on M 37, turn west on 15 Mile Road. Follow Roosevelt Drive northwest 1.5 miles. Turn left; look for signs to direct you to the campground.

GPS COORDINATES   N43° 46.272'   W85° 53.316'

9

Pines Point National Forest Campground

The place is busy on hot summer weekends, as families spend whole days floating around and around—it's nature's own aquatic carousel.

The **White River** begins north of White Cloud in Newaygo County. Fed by swelling groundwater and numerous streams, it flows past farms and small country towns and through the southern portion of the Manistee National Forest. It's a lively river—not too quick and not too wide—with a childlike tendency to wander. Trace the river's path on a map and you will find it winding, resisting the straight line, and in places nearly looping back on itself. In fact, just southwest of Hesperia, a bend in the river forms a stylized U, returning within yards of its original path. The land within this bend is known as Pines Point and gives its name to the greater Pines Point National Forest Recreation Area.

The recreation-area campground has 32 sites on land that sits a bit higher than the nearby White River. Though the campground loosely follows the river's path, only a few sites sit right on the water. The road through the northern part of the campground forms a loop. The choicest sites, in my opinion, are on the right side of the road as you drive into the campground. Sites 7 and 8 directly overlook the water. Though floored with sand and packed dirt, the sites are spacious, level, and free from a lot of undergrowth.

It was long known that Native Americans inhabited this part of the state. During recent renovations at the campground, artifacts were found, and the area next to site 7 has been cordoned off with a split-rail fence, protecting a native cemetery. In fact, the campground host told me about a young man who, a few weeks before my visit, found a spearhead while playing down by the river. This kind of thing is certainly not unheard of in

:: Ratings

BEAUTY: ★ ★ ★ ★ ★
PRIVACY: ★ ★ ★
SPACIOUSNESS: ★ ★ ★ ★ ★
QUIET: ★ ★ ★ ★ ★
SECURITY: ★ ★ ★ ★ ★
CLEANLINESS: ★ ★ ★ ★ ★

:: Key Information

ADDRESS: 650 North Michigan Avenue, Baldwin, MI 49304

OPERATED BY: Huron-Manistee National Forest, Baldwin/White Cloud Ranger District

CONTACT: 231-745-4631; **tinyurl.com/ofgpb2d**

OPEN: Early May–late September

SITES: 32

EACH SITE: Picnic table, fire pit with grill, and lantern post

ASSIGNMENT: First come, first served; reservations can be made online at **recreation.gov.**

REGISTRATION: Self-register at campground.

FACILITIES: Well water, modern restrooms, and vault toilets

PARKING: At site

FEE: $16

ELEVATION: 664 feet

RESTRICTIONS:

■ **Pets:** On leash only

■ **Fires:** Fire pits only

■ **Vehicles:** 2 per site

■ **Other:** 14-day stay limit

western Michigan, but the stories are not as common as they once were.

On the main loop, you will find sites 10–28. Campers access the river by way of a path that runs between sites 13 and 15. Sites along the river here are nice, but those along the back side of the loop don't fill up as fast and offer more seclusion. As at many national-forest recreation areas, the facilities here are top-notch. The campgrounds feature modern restrooms. Sometimes a fancy flush toilet is all it takes to get a reluctant camper excited to spend a weekend in the woods.

Anglers know the White River as a high-quality fly-fishing river—the kind of place you congratulate yourself for discovering. It is Michigan's southernmost trout stream, and many consider it one of the state's best-kept secrets. Fed by cold springs, the water is not overly warmed by a string of dams, and that keeps it at a temperature that allows certain fisheries to thrive. The salmon and trout populations are relatively strong, and the right season offers impressive runs of steelhead.

Hikers have a few options at Pines Point. Old maps and guidebooks make mention of the White River Trail, which is said to follow the river for 12 miles. I've not met anyone in recent years who's been able to pick up on the trailhead. The land south and west of the campground, however, is incorporated into the descriptively named White River Semiprimitive Nonmotorized Recreation Area. You'll find a map for the area at the campground. A great number of the Forest Service roads are open only to foot traffic, and hikers more familiar with the White River SNRA tell me that a trail near the river can be found a little more than a mile south of the campground at FS 9364. This isn't a well-maintained trail with clear blazes, however, so unless you're okay with getting tangled up or lost, I'd stick with the roads.

The point itself is a popular day-use picnic area. A visit to Pines Point for non-campers costs $4 for each vehicle. Walk the trail down to the point from the parking lot, and you immediately understand how this area got its name. The earth is coated in rust-red needles, and at eye level all you see are trunks. Look up and you feel dwarfed by towering pines. According to folks whose families have come here for generations, campers made their way here long before the national forest installed a formal campground,

from places such as Grand Rapids and Muskegon, to pitch tents alongside the river. It's easy to see why.

The loop of the river is the picnic area's biggest draw. Kids can toss an inner tube into the river on one side of the loop, float for 30–40 minutes, and arrive back at the picnic area, just feet from where they put in. The place is busy on hot summer weekends as families spend whole days floating around and around—it's nature's own aquatic carousel.

The river provides recreation for more than just anglers and warm-weather tubers. There are close to 33 miles of excellent paddling on White River from Hesperia to where the water drains into White Lake in Whitehall. An easy three-hour float can be had by putting in upstream in Hesperia and taking out at Pines Point.

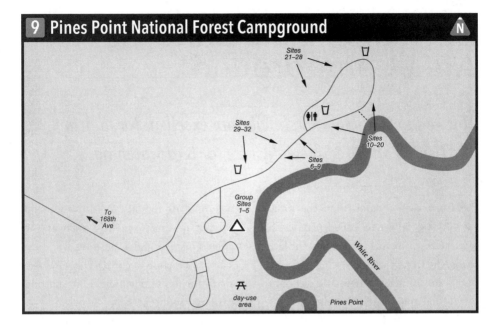

:: Getting There

From Hesperia, drive west on US 20 to 192nd Avenue and turn left. Continue south for a mile to Garfield Road and turn right. Drive west 3 miles to 168th Avenue. The campground is 2.5 miles south of Garfield on 168th.

GPS COORDINATES   N43° 31.812'   W86° 07.020'

10

Haymarsh Lake State Game Area Campground

The wetlands at Haymarsh Lake are excellent for hunting and fishing and are especially nice for bird-watching.

There was a time when the long, shallow lake now called Haymarsh was a series of six smaller lakes. In the late 1940s, the Department of Fish and Game built a concrete dam where a beaver dam once stood and Haymarsh Lake was created. The result is a generally shallow lake (with some deep sections) that has created habitat for a variety of fisheries, attracted waterfowl and songbirds, and served as an anchor for area wildlife. This is, of course, exactly what you want when developing a state game area.

Haymarsh State Game Area attracts hunters and anglers from all over the state. The great variety of birds also attracts bird-watchers. The DNR recommends the site for those looking to spot nesting songbirds, such as the golden-winged and mourning warblers. There is a section of cut-over aspen forest that provides opportunities for spotting various woodpeckers.

The sites at the Haymarsh Game Area Campground are scattered loosely along a mile of the lake's western shore. There are 19 sites in all, and with the exception of the first 5, they are spaced widely, offering campers the most private camping you will find outside a dispersed campground like Nordhouse Dunes. The first set of campsites is close to the entrance on a side road that bends toward the water and then returns to the main route. Sites 1–4 are next to the lake. Site 5 sits on the inside across from 4.

As you drive into the campground, you will notice that the terrain is rather low—many would call it marshy. There is high ground, but in between these dry patches are pocket ponds and wetland. The sites themselves are all on dry ground, but each is surrounded by some of the best mosquito breeding habitat in

:: Ratings

BEAUTY: ★ ★ ★ ★
PRIVACY: ★ ★ ★ ★ ★
SPACIOUSNESS: ★ ★ ★ ★ ★
QUIET: ★ ★ ★ ★
SECURITY: ★ ★ ★ ★
CLEANLINESS: ★ ★ ★ ★

:: Key Information

ADDRESS: 22090 Northland Drive, Paris, MI 49338

OPERATED BY: Mecosta County Parks - Paris Park

CONTACT: 231-796-3420; **www.mecostacountyparks.com /haymarsh.html**

OPEN: Mid-April–February (weather permitting)

SITES: 19

EACH SITE: Picnic table, fire pit, trash can, lantern post

ASSIGNMENT: First come, first served

REGISTRATION: Self-register at campground.

FACILITIES: Hand-pumped water and vault toilets

PARKING: At site

FEE: $13

ELEVATION: 1,058 feet

RESTRICTIONS:

■ **Pets:** On leash only; limited to 2 per site

■ **Fires:** Fire pits only

■ **Vehicles:** 2 per site

the county. Throughout the warm season, come prepared for bugs.

There are just two pit toilets at Haymarsh. The first is located between sites 6 and 7. The second is found at the end of the road, past site 19, near the boat launch parking area. A hand pump for water is located between sites 12 and 13.

My favorite site is 11. A small, lily pad–covered inlet creates a point, and site 11 sits at the end of this point with views north and south down the lake. Farther than most from the road, it also provides more privacy from neighbors—though most sites here are very private. During my last visit here, we watched a blue heron stand motionless a dozen yards away. It eventually took wing and seemed to skim the water as it flew to its next perch.

Campers who come to Haymarsh for the hunting and fishing rarely leave

disappointed. There are no posted trails for hikers, but there are miles of dirt roads crisscrossing the game area, which is itself nearly 6,000 acres. There are also unmarked trails. Hikers taking these paths are advised to bring a compass and map, and to know how to use them.

For other recreation, you will have to leave the campground. The nearby town of Big Rapids is perhaps best known as the home of Ferris State University. You might hear rumors of the campus being a bit rowdy during the school year, but in the summer, Big Rapids is a quiet town. Michigan's second longest river, the Muskegon, flows north to south through town on its way to Lake Michigan. One of the most enjoyable ways to spend an afternoon in the area is a long float down the Muskegon River on a tube. The activity is so popular, and so many people can

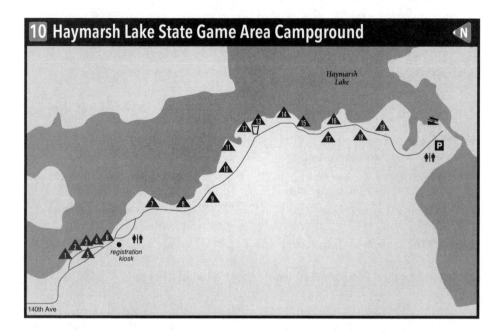

be seen floating by on warm summer days, that Big Rapids broadly proclaims itself as The Tubing Capital of Michigan. If you have any interest, head over to Sawmill Tube & Canoe Livery (231-796-6408; sawmillmi.com) on Baldwin Street, right on the river. They have sent nearly half a million people down the river and really know what they're about. Keep in mind that when the water is running high, the two-hour float trip can be half as long—in which case, I would recommend the longer trip.

:: Getting There

From US 131, just north of Big Rapids, take Exit 142 for 19 Mile Road. Head east 1.8 miles to Northland Road. Turn left and continue north 2.5 miles. Then head east on Hoover Road. The main route through follows Hoover, 180th Avenue, and 21 Mile Road for 7.4 miles. To miss a turn would be hard to do. When 21 Mile Road bends to the north, turn right on 140th Avenue. Follow this less than a half mile to the end of the road and the entrance to the campground.

GPS COORDINATES N43° 45.719' W85° 21.670'

11

Tubbs Lake State Forest Campgrounds

Situated on a small island accessed by a narrow strip of land that passes through cattails, purple loosestrifes, and pickerel-weed, these campgrounds are wonderfully secluded.

E **arly in** the 1900s, a beaver dam first gave the Martiny Lakes in northeastern Mecosta County their shape. In 1955, the Michigan Department of Natural Resources made the flooding more or less permanent with the construction of Winchester Dam. The dam raised water levels 8 feet, creating a chain of eight interconnected lakes: Big Evans, Manake, Saddlebag, Bullhead, Boom, Dogfish, Lost, and Tubbs. (The tally of lakes varies, depending on who's counting. The number gets confused by people who include Pretty Lake and Diamond Lake in the mix.)

Most of these small lakes are only 25–30 feet deep, and the places where they connect are shallow and surrounded by wetlands. On Tubbs Lake in particular, the overall shallowness is a boon, the waters providing a home to a stand of wild rice. This plant, which was much used by Native Americans, grows only in the Great Lakes region of the country, but most stands are found in the Upper Peninsula, northern Wisconsin, and Minnesota. In recent years, faculty from Ferris State University in nearby Big Rapids have led a four-day Wild Rice Camp in early September on Tubbs Lake. Participants learn how to make their own wooden tools for harvesting; how to collect, store, and prepare the rice; and how to reseed and restore wild-rice populations at other locations.

The two campgrounds on Tubbs Lake are part of Pere Marquette State Forest, and both are operated by Mecosta County Parks. Each campground offers sites on the water and easy boat access for getting out on the lake. The most interesting of the pair is the Tubbs Island Campground. Situated on a small island

:: Ratings

BEAUTY: ★ ★ ★ ★
PRIVACY: ★ ★ ★ ★
SPACIOUSNESS: ★ ★ ★ ★ ★
QUIET: ★ ★ ★ ★
SECURITY: ★ ★ ★ ★
CLEANLINESS: ★ ★ ★ ★ ★

:: Key Information

ADDRESS: 22250 Northland Drive, Paris, MI 49332

OPERATED BY: Mecosta County Parks

CONTACT: 989-382-7158; **mecosta countyparks.com/tubbslake.html**

OPEN: April–mid-October

SITES: 33

EACH SITE: Picnic table and fire pit

ASSIGNMENT: First come, first served

REGISTRATION: Self-register at campground.

FACILITIES: Hand-pumped water and vault toilets

PARKING: At site only

FEE: $15

ELEVATION: 1,011 feet

RESTRICTIONS:

■ **Pets:** On leash only

■ **Fires:** Fire pits only

■ **Alcohol:** Permitted

accessed by a narrow strip of land that passes through cattails, purple loosestrifes, and pickerelweed, this campground is wonderfully secluded. Across the way, campers will still see boats along the shore, cottages here and there, and the hard-to-ignore Tubbs Lake Resort (a private campground easily recognized by the rows of RVs and fifth-wheel trailers), but the island offers a sense of privacy that's much appreciated by campers.

Tubbs Island Campground has 12 sites, all but 2 of which are on the water. Sites 1–7 are on the high end of the island and overlook the lake. Sites 1–3 face the lake's more open water. Sites 8–10, near the low side, offer semiobstructed views of the water, which is blocked by trees and, in the case of 10, cattails and such.

Personally, I prefer the two walk-in sites, 11 and 12. Campers looking for a little more isolation will drive the one-way loop around the campground and find, just as the loop ends, a small area for parking on the left. From there, it's a short hike up the hill to one of the two sites. Though not right on the water, both sit high on the wooded hill, overlooking the lake.

The Martiny Chain of Lakes is fed by Chippewa Creek, which flows into Saddlebag Lake at the west end of the flooding. It exits over the Winchester Dam in the east as the Chippewa River, eventually flowing into the Tittabawassee, which empties into the Saginaw, which in turn empties into Saginaw Bay near Bay City. The eastern arm of Tubbs Lake stretches due east from Tubbs Island, around a final promontory—which is also where to find the Tubbs Lake Mainland Campground. (By road, simply get back on Madison Road heading east. Turn left on Birch Haven Drive and follow the signs.)

The mainland campground is laid out like a strand of Christmas lights, with a small loop of six sites at the end. More than half of the campground's 21 sites look out over the water. Sites 1–9 are set back a little in the woods. Site 10 is half woods with some waterfront. During our last visit, I regretted not being able to pitch our tent on site 11 or 12—both were very picturesque.

Surrounded by 1,600 acres of the Martiny Lake State Game Area, a property full of woods and wetlands, the region is considered a sportsman's paradise by many regulars. The lakes are dotted with boat launches, and the game area encompasses more bodies of water than just those of the lake chain. Bluegill, Bass, Mud, and Half-Moon Lakes all abut at least a portion of this retreat for hunters and anglers. (Duck hunting is also popular here.)

Farther downstream, closer to Mount Pleasant, the Chippewa River is popular with tubers, but paddlers jump in not far from here. Just about 7 miles northeast, a dam in Barryton collects the west and north branches of the river. Paddlers put in at the dam and enjoy more than 80 miles of picturesque canoeing. But there's really no need to go so far a-paddle to enjoy some time on the water. An entire day could be spent fishing or simply exploring the Martiny Lakes, and even more if you ventured into nearby Pretty Lake or Jehnsen Lake.

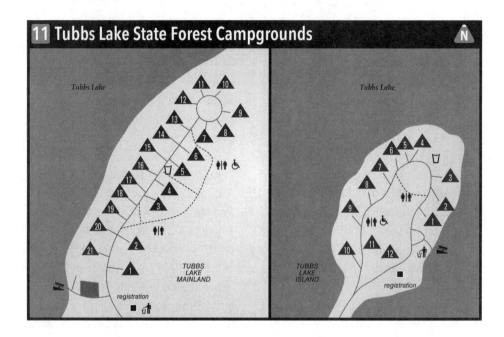

:: Getting There

Coming from the west, follow M 20 east out of Big Rapids. Fourteen miles out, turn left on 80th Avenue and follow that north to Taft. Turn right on Taft, then left on 65th Avenue, and follow that around as it turns into Madison Road. From the east, follow M 20 west out of Mount Pleasant. Turn north on M 66. After 8 miles, turn west on 17 Mile Road. The first left is 45th Avenue; turn south, and in a half mile head west again on Madison Road. Once you're on Madison, signs will direct you to the campgrounds.

GPS COORDINATES   N43° 42.834'   W85° 12.624'

Northwest Michigan

●●●●●●●●●●●●●●

12

Ludington State Park:
JACK PINE WALK-IN CAMPGROUND

This campground rewards you with quiet nights, where all you hear is the sound of waves on Lake Michigan.

Ask **Michiganders** their favorite place to camp, and you're likely to hear Ludington State Park more often than not. It's hard to overestimate the popularity of this 5,300-acre recreation destination nestled between Hamlin Lake and Lake Michigan. The park consistently earns top spots on the annual lists of Michigan's most popular attractions, best beaches, and favorite campgrounds.

Most visitors park alongside the drive up into the park, hoof it over the foredune, and lay out their towels, coolers, and umbrellas on one of the most beautiful stretches of Lake Michigan beach. Others venture farther in. The river that empties Hamlin Lake into Lake Michigan sees a regular parade of inner-tubers

:: Ratings

BEAUTY: ★ ★ ★ ★ ★
PRIVACY: ★ ★ ★ ★ ★
SPACIOUSNESS: ★ ★ ★ ★ ★
QUIET: ★ ★ ★ ★ ★
SECURITY: ★ ★ ★
CLEANLINESS: ★ ★ ★ ★ ★

floating from one lake to the other, then walking back through the park to put in on this side of the Hamlin Dam. The more adventurous try hiking and perhaps take the back trails to the Big Sable Point Lighthouse.

The park has three modern campgrounds—Pines, Cedars, and Beechwood. Among campgrounds packed with RVs, fifth-wheel trailers, pop-ups, and the occasional tent mansions, these aren't bad at all. The campgrounds conform to the interesting contours of the land, and this creates space for unique sites. Several years back, you would have found my tent pitched somewhere in the Beechwood Campground, perhaps at site 232 between the first two loops. There are a few choice sites like this one, somewhat set apart and close to Lost Lake.

Today, however, you would find me hauling my gear on my back to the Jack Pine Walk-In Campground. Ten sites on two spurs are hunkered down in the sand behind the park's long foredune. To get there, campers have to follow Lighthouse Trail (essentially a sidewalk) a mile up

:: Key Information

ADDRESS: 8800 West M 116, Ludington, MI 49431

OPERATED BY: Michigan DNR-Ludington State Park

CONTACT: 231-843-2423; **michigan.gov/ludington**

OPEN: Year-round

SITES: 10

EACH SITE: Picnic table and fire pit

ASSIGNMENT: Reservations can be made online at **midnrreservations.com** and by calling 800-447-2757.

REGISTRATION: Register at campground registration building on M 116 as you drive into the park.

FACILITIES: Hand-pumped water and pit toilets

PARKING: Lot near park entrance

FEE: $16 ($12 off-season)

ELEVATION: 590 feet

RESTRICTIONS:

■ **Pets:** On leash only (and not near the water)

■ **Fires:** Fire pits only

■ **Alcohol:** Permitted

■ **Vehicles:** Michigan Recreation Passport required

the beach from the Pines Campground. You're free to use wagons, bikes, or even a wheelbarrow, if that's what you need, but vehicles are prohibited.

With the exception of jack pines and some juniper bushes, there is little vegetation, just dune grass and some frost grapevines. The first spur, sites A–E, is more out in the open. Buried in a cluster of stunted pine trees, site E is the exception. It sits across the way from the other four sites and offers a private retreat, somewhat protected from the sun and wind. More shade can be found at site F on the campground's other spur. Bushes and low trees screen the remaining sites, G–J, from each other, but not so much from the sun.

This campground requires some extra work on the part of visitors. The

park defines quiet hours at Jack Pine as "all the time" but "especially between 11 p.m. and 8 a.m.," and campers have to bag out their own trash and leave it in Dumpsters near the park entrance. The campground repays the attention with quiet nights, where all you hear is the sound of waves on Lake Michigan.

From the walk-in campground, you are already halfway to Big Sable Point Lighthouse, via Lighthouse Trail. This is the sister light to the Little Sable Lighthouse in Silver Lake, about 35 miles south of here. Built back in 1867, the tower was originally constructed of yellow brick. A few decades later, the brick began to crumble, and the lighthouse was reinforced with iron bands and concrete wrapped around its exterior. The work on the light required it to be painted. The black-and-white stripes you see today were chosen to make the lighthouse more visible during the day. For a small donation, visitors can climb the tower, but if you really want to experience life in a lighthouse, ask about the volunteer keeper program.

The lighthouse served many years guiding ships around the Grande Pointe au Sable but was apparently too little help for the George F. Foster, a schooner bound for Chicago with a load of lumber. The ship was blown ashore by a gale in the fall of 1872. You can explore the wreck, for what it is, without even getting your feet wet. The ship is right up on shore, not too far south of the Jack Pine Walk-In Campground. It is almost entirely buried by beach sand, but the park has thoughtfully marked off the ship's dimensions and posted an informative sign.

The hike out to the lighthouse is an easy, level, 2-mile walk from the main parking lot via the beach or the aforementioned Lighthouse Trail. A more roundabout path takes you into the heart of the park along the Lighthouse Trail. All told, Ludington State Park has 21.5 miles of trails offering a variety of experiences. To escape the beach, try hiking out along the Island Trail, which begins by traversing the chain of small islands that define Lost Lake and then follows the western edge of Hamlin Lake. Return via the Ridge and Lost Lake trails. For a short hike, head over to the visitor center. The Skyline Trail there climbs to the top of the dunes and follows a boardwalk along the high ridge.

For something altogether unique, Ludington State Park has a defined canoe trail. Boats can be rented there at the park, or you can bring your own. With paddle in hand, you put in at the boat launch near Hamlin Dam and follow the shoreline south. Several coves and channels keep the route interesting. Most of the park that you see from the water here is inaccessible to cars and foot traffic.

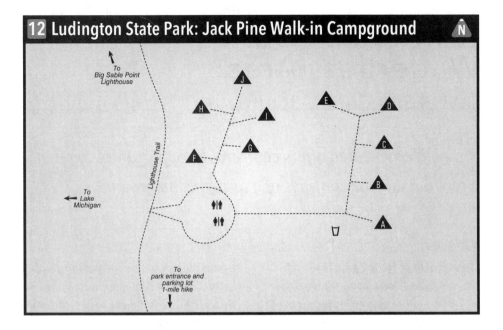

:: Getting There

From Ludington, follow US 10 into town and turn right (north) on North Lakeshore Drive. In about 2.5 miles, you come to a fork in the road. Continue to the left on M 116; the park is 4 miles ahead at the end of the road.

GPS COORDINATES   N44° 02.664'   W86° 30.684'

13

Nordhouse Dunes Wilderness Area:

DISPERSED CAMPGROUND

This wilderness area offers campers the opportunity to pitch a tent outside the confines of a formal campground.

In 1987, Congress passed the Michigan Wilderness Act, which identified regions within Michigan's national forests that were worthy of being restored to a natural state. The law created 10 wilderness areas that have changed the state's landscape, so to speak, for those who appreciate an unspoiled experience of nature. Today, more than 30 years later, not everyone has heard of the Horseshoe Bay Wilderness or the Big Island Lake Wilderness, but it's hard to imagine a Michigan without the Upper Peninsula's Sylvania Wilderness Area or the Lower Peninsula's Nordhouse Dunes.

:: Ratings

BEAUTY: ★ ★ ★ ★
PRIVACY: ★ ★ ★ ★ ★
SPACIOUSNESS: ★ ★ ★ ★ ★
QUIET: ★ ★ ★ ★
SECURITY: ★ ★ ★ ★ ★
CLEANLINESS: ★ ★ ★ ★ ★

The Nordhouse Dunes Wilderness Area is the only such wilderness area in the Lower Peninsula. Composed of 3,450 acres, the park shares a border with Ludington State Park to the south and with the Manistee National Forest to the north and east. The preserve's fourth boundary is 4 miles of undeveloped Lake Michigan shoreline. This wilderness area offers campers the opportunity to hike and explore the coastal dune regions of Lake Michigan, as well as to pitch a tent outside the confines of a formal campground (the U.S. Forest Service calls it dispersed camping).

I would recommend getting a good trail guide before diving into the Nordhouse Dunes. *Backpacking in Michigan* by Jim DuFresne is an excellent resource and describes 50 excellent places to backpack in the state, including the Nordhouse Dunes. For the purpose of this book, I will simply offer a bare sketch of one of many possible itineraries.

There are two main trailheads into the dunes. From the north, campers

:: Key Information

ADDRESS: 412 Red Apple Road, Mio, MI 49660

OPERATED BY: Huron-Manistee National Forest, Cadillac/Manistee Ranger District

CONTACT: 231-723-2211; tinyurl.com/2eyupsd

OPEN: Year-round, though not maintained in winter

SITES: n/a

EACH SITE: n/a

ASSIGNMENT: First come, first served

REGISTRATION: Self-register at campground.

FACILITIES: Vault toilets at trailheads

PARKING: Trailhead parking areas

FEE: No fee for camping in wilderness; $5/day vehicle fee for parking at trailhead, $15/week

ELEVATION: 653 feet

RESTRICTIONS:

■ **Pets:** On leash only

■ **Fires:** Not permitted on beaches; collecting woody material from beaches or sandy areas is prohibited.

■ **Vehicles:** All motorized vehicles prohibited

■ **Other:** Campsites should be at least 400 feet from Lake Michigan, 250 feet from trails and Nordhouse Lake, and 450 feet from developed recreation area.

access the trails from the Lake Michigan Recreation Area. From the south, there's a parking area and trailhead at the end of Nurnberg Road. Near the northern trailhead, a 122-step climb takes you to the top of an observation tower with breathtaking views of Lake Michigan. (Well, I am sure the climb contributes a little to the lack of breath, but the view from up top is nevertheless outstanding.) The wilderness trails here no longer have names, but those familiar with the dunes might remember the route that was once known as the Michigan Trail. From the north, the old Michigan Trail runs south, parallel to the shore, for about 2 miles. The route features a nice walk over ancient dunes, straddling the line between forest and open sand.

Eventually, the path leads inland and takes you to the southern trailhead, where you can find a path back to the recreation area to complete a 6-mile loop.

Dunes are forever evolving. Not only does the wind constantly shape the contours of the sand closest to the lake, but farther inland, where the older portions of the dunes lie, you can also find nature transforming the shifting sands to stable forest. From sandy hills to woods stocked with beeches, sugar maples, red and white oaks, and such evergreens as red and white pines, Nordhouse Dunes is a hands-on lesson in ecology.

The rules for camping in the dunes are fairly simple. You must camp more than 400 feet from the Lake Michigan shoreline, 250 feet from established trails and Nordhouse Lake, and 450 feet from the recreation area. You are asked not to camp anywhere that signs indicate no camping, and one rule states that visitors shall not be naked in public. Aside from that, camp where you will and how you will. I would suggest, however, that setting up on the open dunes will lead to more sand in your tent, hair, and clothes than you can imagine. I prefer to seek the shelter of some trees.

Most campers will approach the dunes from US 31, making the final drive in on West Forest Trail Road or Nurnberg Road. The former, as the name suggests, leads to the campground and day-use area. The latter leads to the southern parking area and trailhead. Connecting the two, Green Road parallels, but sits just outside, the wilderness's eastern boundary. Along this narrow, sandy Forest Service road, three unofficial primitive sites offer visitors a convenient and rather secluded escape. The sites are bare-bones—no picnic tables, no sources of drinkable water, and no outhouses. A few have rudimentary

pit toilets of the open-air-throne variety, but the nearest proper vault toilet is at the trailhead on Nurnberg Road.

Green Road is rough, but people find it possible to get small trailers onto these sites. With just three campsites spread out over a mile or so, there's plenty of room to spread out and lots of privacy. Typical of the dunes ecology, the sites are sandy, with dune grass growing in patches. Beeches and some evergreens provide shade, and, where the terrain falls away into lower land behind the campsites, the ground is blanketed in ferns.

For more traditional car camping, consider a stay at the Lake Michigan Recreation Area Campground. This national-forest campground offers 99 sites on four loops, flush toilets, and direct trail access to the wilderness. The day-use area has a popular beach on Lake Michigan, bike trails, a playground, and a few nice hiking loops. This campground fills up in the summer (especially weekends), so consider reservations. Only some sites can be reserved; the rest are yours on a first-come, first-serve basis.

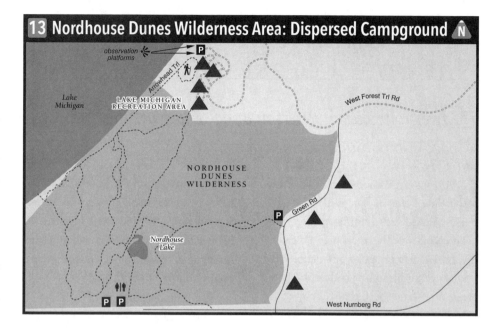

:: Getting There

The wilderness area is located between Ludington and Manistee, west of US 31. From the north, take US 31 south to West County Line Road. Drive west to Quarter-line Road, head south 3.2 miles to West Forest Trail Road, and turn west. The Lake Michigan Recreation Area is 5 miles in. From points south, take US 31 to West Forest Trail Road, turn left (west), and drive 7.6 miles to the recreation area.

GPS COORDINATES   N44° 07.074'   W86° 24.864'

14

Peterson Bridge South National Forest Campground

The riverfront sites at Peterson Bridge South are this wooded campground's hidden gems.

If **you** have taken canoe trips down the Pine River in the past, especially one organized by an outfitter, there is a good chance you have been to Peterson Bridge. There is a popular put-in north of the bridge for groups of paddlers. There are several large outfitters nearby (The Pine River Paddlesports Center, Horina's Canoe and Kayak Rental, and just up the road apiece, Bosman's Pine River Canoe Rental), and they regularly drop off adventurers ready to tackle the river.

The put-in is directly across from the campground. The camp manager told me on my last visit that it's actually quite entertaining to sit on the bluff overlooking the put-in when a group first sets out. There are always a few people who have never been on the water in a canoe before, and inevitably they get all turned around trying to find their balance. At least a handful of canoes will flip and dump their passengers before they get even a hundred feet down the river.

The campground itself is a bit of a surprise. Drive through and you will count only 20 sites. Because this is a National Forest campground, the road is paved. There is a brightly lit bathroom in the center of the campground with drinking fountains, sinks, and flush toilets. There are additional vault toilets distributed throughout the camp. If this were all there is to Peterson Bridge, it would be a fine campground, but there's so much more. After leaving your car at the parking area near the registration kiosk, you'll take a path leading down to the river. This is the route to the campground's 11 walk- or paddle-in campsites.

The first campsite as you walk is located on a rise overlooking the water. From this vantage point, campers can look across and down at the public put-in on the other side of the water. Continuing to walk alongside the river, heading

:: Ratings

BEAUTY: ★ ★ ★ ★ ★
PRIVACY: ★ ★ ★ ★
SPACIOUSNESS: ★ ★ ★ ★ ★
QUIET: ★ ★ ★ ★
SECURITY: ★ ★ ★ ★ ★
CLEANLINESS: ★ ★ ★ ★ ★

:: Key Information

ADDRESS: 1755 South Mitchell Street, Cadillac, MI 49601

OPERATED BY: Huron-Manistee National Forest, Baldwin/White Cloud Ranger District

CONTACT: 231-745-4631; tinyurl.com/q374y7q

OPEN: Year-round, maintained May–October

SITES: 31

EACH SITE: Picnic table, fire pit, lantern post

ASSIGNMENT: First come, first served

REGISTRATION: Self-register at campground.

FACILITIES: Vault toilets, modern restroom (no showers), drinking water

PARKING: At site (or near entrance for walk-in sites)

FEE: $18 ($6/person for walk-in tent sites)

ELEVATION: 838 feet

RESTRICTIONS:

- **Pets:** On leash only
- **Fires:** Fire pits only
- **Vehicles:** 2 per site
- **Other:** 14-day stay limit

upstream, the path enters a quiet pocket of woods—northern cedars, oak, and maple, mostly. The forest floor is covered in ferns, and two campsites are set here back against the bottom of the bluff.

Leaving the woods, the path ends at a sandy beach on the Pine River. This is where paddlers exit the river if they need a campsite for the night. For their convenience, there is a self-registration kiosk here, as well as drinking water. On either side of the sandy boat area are two campsites. Six more sit farther back—though the river bends around and two of these sites are close to the water.

The brush around these sites is full of poison ivy, so I wouldn't recommend tramping through the weeds. But the sites themselves are plenty spacious and

well trimmed, so there's no real chance of accidentally stumbling into the noxious ivy.

The river is so close here that you can hear it flowing as you drift off to sleep at night. They say that flowing water creates negative ions, and negative ions are believed to help increase levels of serotonin in the body, helping to relieve stress and boost energy. If this is true, and the science plays out, there's all the more reason to haul all that gear down to the river for some camping.

From these riverfront campsites, a stairway leads up the hill to the main campground. Halfway up you will pass a set of vault toilets, but continue to the top, and the modern restrooms are just a stone's throw away. If the camp managers

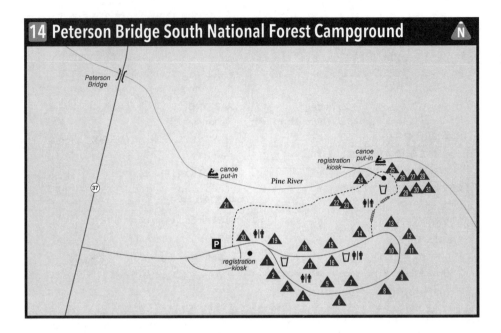

at Peterson Bridge continue to be as amiable as they have been in the past, you can always ask if they can drive you down to the tent sites in the camp golf cart.

A short drive to the south is the Pine River Paddlesports Center. In addition to outfitting families and groups for trips on the Pine River, the center maintains a private campground. Created with tent-camping families in mind, the campground has established a few rules to ensure guests have a positive experience—in particular, no pets, no fireworks, no loud music, and no foul language. While Peterson Bridge is generally a quiet place to camp, one bad apple can spoil the lot. It's not likely you'll have loud, obnoxious neighbors, but if you do, moving to the private campground might save you the disappointment of heading home early.

:: Getting There

From US 131, take Exit 176 for M 115/M 55 west. Stay on M 55 when the roads split in 3 miles. Continue west on M 55 for 18 miles to the four-way stop at M 37. Turn south. Peterson Bridge is 1.5 miles from the intersection. The campground is on the east side of the road just south of the bridge.

GPS COORDINATES   N44° 12.117'   W85° 48.098'

15

Silver Creek State Forest Campground

For hiking and paddling, the campground at the confluence of the Pine River and Silver Creek is just the thing.

The **Pine River** runs through a number of counties—Osceola, Lake, Wexford, and Manistee. From Edgett's Bridge (about 6.5 miles east-northeast of Luther) to the Low Bridge takeout, the river offers 60 miles of canoeing and fishing. A combination of fast water and easy accessibility made the Pine very popular—so popular, in fact, that before the U.S. Forest Service restricted the number of boats on the water, summer could see 2,000 canoes making the run every week. Visit the Pine River, and you'll understand the fuss. You'll also appreciate not seeing so many canoes on the water these days.

A couple of campgrounds get you close to the river. The Peterson Bridge South Campground is one. Right off M 37, Peterson Bridge is maintained by the U.S. Forest Service. It has flush toilets and drinking water. Farther upstream, the Michigan Department of Natural Resources operates the Lincoln Bridge State Forest Campground. Even farther upstream, where Silver Creek empties into the Pine, is the incomparable Silver Creek State Forest Campground.

The campground offers a mix of campsites. On the main loop, there are 19 sites perfect for tents and small trailers. The lots are well manicured, and benches overlook the picturesque Pine River as it flows by. The best of the lot, however, are the seven walk-in sites located on a long, narrow bend in the river. These are spacious and offer plenty of solitude, close enough to the water for you to be lulled to sleep by the sound.

An interesting adventure around the Pine River can be had by hiking or biking the 4-mile Silver Creek Pathway. The pathway passes right through the campground, entering near site 10 and leaving

:: Ratings

BEAUTY: ★ ★ ★ ★
PRIVACY: ★ ★ ★ ★
SPACIOUSNESS: ★ ★ ★ ★ ★
QUIET: ★ ★ ★ ★
SECURITY: ★ ★ ★ ★ ★
CLEANLINESS: ★ ★ ★ ★ ★

:: Key Information

ADDRESS: 2468 West 24th Street, Baldwin, MI 49304

OPERATED BY: Michigan DNR-Baldwin Field Office

CONTACT: 231-745-9465; **tinyurl.com/mxpg8jg**

OPEN: Year-round, maintained May–October

SITES: 26

EACH SITE: Picnic table, fire pit

ASSIGNMENT: First come, first served

REGISTRATION: Self-register at campground.

FACILITIES: Hand-pumped water and vault toilets

PARKING: At site (parking area for walk-in sites)

FEE: $13

ELEVATION: 950 feet

RESTRICTIONS:

■ **Pets:** On leash only

■ **Fires:** Fire pits only

■ **Vehicles:** 2 per site; Michigan Recreation Passport required

■ **Other:** 14-day stay limit

by way of a scenic bridge over the Pine River. It continues up one side of the river, and back down the other. The loop is kept separate from the area's off-road-vehicle trails, though you might hear the whine of motors echo through the woods from time to time.

A chief reason to camp at the Silver Creek campground is the Pine River. A significant tributary of the Manistee, the Pine has a solid reputation in the state among paddlers and anglers. Paddlers come for the 7% river grade, which makes this the fastest-flowing water (on average) in the Lower Peninsula. Fast runs and tight turns and some Class I and II rapids thrill beginning paddlers, giving them stories to tell later on of that time they faced down

real danger and lived to paddle another day. And depending on how green you are when it comes to paddling, the river can be a challenge and shouldn't be taken lightly. But experienced whitewater canoers and kayakers will find the ride to be more of an obstacle course than a roller coaster. Scattered boulders and seasonal tree falls add to the negotiations.

Designated a National Wild and Scenic River, the Pine takes you deep into the national forest. Surrounded by cedars, mixed hardwoods, and pines, you can easily lose yourself in the experience—that is, when you're not watching the river for the next banked turn. While the entire 20-plus-mile run from Silver Creek would leave paddlers on the water for a good part of the day (likely more than eight hours), you're never more than about 4 or 5 miles from the next access point, road, or bridge.

The Pine is also an official Blue Ribbon Trout Stream. This honor is bestowed on rivers for their quality of water, their accessibility, and the ability of fishery to support itself through natural reproduction. The Pine has some of the coldest water among Lower Peninsula rivers. Trout love it, and fly rods and fishing line should be included among the obstacles paddlers have to deal with.

Between May 15 and September 30, the U.S. Forest Service requires a watercraft permit for boats on the Pine River Corridor. The corridor begins at Elm Flats and ends at the Low Bridge Landing, just before the river enters Tippy Pond. You don't need a vehicle pass at nearby Lincoln Bridge, but all access points downstream are within the protected stretch of river, and you'll need a USFS vehicle pass. The watercraft permits are free, though there's a $2 reservation fee, and I wouldn't count on getting a permit without a reservation. They can be reserved by calling, visiting, or sending a letter to the Baldwin/White Cloud Ranger Station or the Cadillac/Manistee Ranger Station.

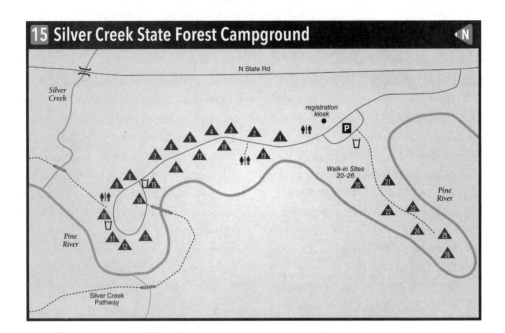

:: Getting There

From Baldwin, take M 37 north 11 miles to Hermit Road (aka Old M 63). Turn east. Drive 8 miles to North State Road, and turn left. Drive 4 miles north just shy of East 9 Mile Road. The campground is right there on the west side. The signs are pretty clear. If you come to Lincoln Bridge State Forest Campground, you've gone a mile too far.

GPS COORDINATES   N44° 06.878'   W85° 41.005'

16

CCC Bridge State Forest Campground

Even if your plans don't include a canoe, kayak, or inner tube, a quiet spot along the Manistee River shouldn't be overlooked.

It's intriguing to realize how close the Au Sable and Manistee Rivers in northern Michigan are to each other on the map. Both originate just south of Gaylord, run a parallel path south, and suddenly part near Grayling—the Au Sable eventually finding Lake Huron; the Manistee, Lake Michigan. Lake Margrethe, west of Grayling, was once known as Portage Lake, a name that is still attached to its creek, which empties into the Manistee. On a good map, you can see why. Old-time travelers crossing Michigan's Lower Peninsula would have found the several-mile portage from the Au Sable to Lake Margrethe an easy alternative to paddling around the tip of the mitt. In

fact, long-distance paddlers still tackle the 270-mile route today.

The Au Sable River is the more popular of the two in this part of the state, but I suspect that has more to do with easy accessibility in Grayling than a comparison of each river's qualities. The Upper Manistee is protected as part of the Michigan Natural Rivers Program, while the Lower Manistee has been designated a National Wild and Scenic River. All told, the river enjoys a fine reputation among paddlers and anglers, and you will regularly see hordes of kids floating by camp in tubes. Two canoe liveries, one in Grayling and another in Kalkaska (see Key Information), offer trips that cover most of this upper portion of the river.

The CCC Bridge is the perfect spot for a campground. Thru-paddlers, of course, appreciate any nice place to stop for the night. Day-trippers putting in near M 72 in Grayling will find, 5–7 hours later, the CCC Bridge waiting in the distance. A parking lot at the entrance to the south campground serves paddlers and tubers,

:: Ratings

BEAUTY: ★ ★ ★ ★
PRIVACY: ★ ★ ★
SPACIOUSNESS: ★ ★ ★ ★
QUIET: ★ ★ ★
SECURITY: ★ ★ ★ ★
CLEANLINESS: ★ ★ ★ ★ ★

:: Key Information

ADDRESS: 1132 US 31, Traverse City, MI 49686

OPERATED BY: Traverse City State Park

CONTACT: 231-922-5270; **tinyurl.com/369df2p.** Canoe liveries on the Manistee include Shel-Haven Canoe and Kayak Rental in Grayling (989-348-2158; **shelhaven.com**) and Long's Canoe Livery in Kalkaska (989-348-7224 or 231-258-3452; **longscanoelivery.com**).

OPEN: Year-round, though snow may prevent access

SITES: 31

EACH SITE: Picnic table and fire pit

ASSIGNMENT: First come, first served

REGISTRATION: Self-register at campground.

FACILITIES: Hand-pumped water and vault toilets

PARKING: At site

FEE: $13

ELEVATION: 1,082 feet

RESTRICTIONS:

■ **Pets:** On leash only

■ **Fires:** Fire pits only

■ **Alcohol:** Permitted

■ **Vehicles:** Michigan Recreation Passport required

and vans arrive pretty regularly, especially on weekends, to pull groups from the water. But even if your plans don't include a canoe, kayak, or inner tube, a quiet spot along the Manistee River shouldn't be overlooked. Its humble scenic charms are worth a stay.

As the campground is designed for campers with tents and small trailers, bigger rigs tend to find other places to set up. The campground straddles the river at CCC Bridge. North of the bridge, a small outpost of seven sites lies along a single road with a turnaround at the end. Of these, site 4 is the only one not on the river. Separated by a road, a river, and the bridge, the north campground is the quieter of the two. The sites here are grassy, and the river is seen easily through the trees.

The south campground has the other 24 sites. Thirteen of them can be found

on three loops that follow the contour of the water. The land behind the first loop (sites 9–13) seemed boggy on my last visit. Farther along, the second loop (sites 14–18) is on higher ground. A pathway from behind 17 and 18 leads down to the river. Views of the river here are harder to come by, even though the water is flowing just beyond the trees.

The remaining sites lie along a spur to the south of camp. Nestled in pinewoods, the sites here are lined with packed dirt and the reddish hue of pine needles. These sites are the farthest from the water, and, during the height of mosquito season, this might offer some respite from the buzzing horde.

Upstream from CCC Bridge, the state maintains several campgrounds—Lake Margrethe (just south of where the lake flows into Portage Creek), Manistee River

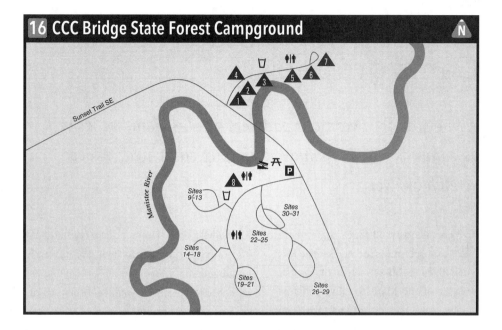

16 CCC Bridge State Forest Campground

Bridge (near M 72), and Upper Manistee River. Like CCC Bridge, they all offer rustic facilities: water from a hand pump and vault toilets.

You can find the headwaters of the Manistee north of the Upper Manistee Campground near the ghost town of Deward in the 4,700-acre Deward Tract, which is part of the Au Sable State Forest. The tract features the state's only Pine Stump Preserve—42.5 acres that have been set aside to "protect the evidence of early logging efforts in Michigan" (as described by the Michigan Department of Natural Resources).

The water between M 72 and CCC Bridge is prime fly-fishing water. In fact, that's the only fishing allowed here. The warm-water fishery at Lake Margrethe supports a fine population of smallmouth bass and muskies, but the cold Manistee is all about the trout. Anglers will tell you that this river produces some of the largest trout you will ever catch on a fly.

:: Getting There

From Grayling, follow M 72 west. Here, you are actually on M 72 and M 93 at the same time, but M 93 splits off to the south about 1.5 miles out of town. You want to follow M 93 (also called Military Road). About 14 miles down you come to Sunset Trail Road. Turn right (north). The river and the campground are just 1.8 miles up the road.

GPS COORDINATES   N44° 36.846'   W84° 59.436'

17

Baxter Bridge State Forest Campground

A fine stop for overnight paddlers on the Manistee, as well as campers who just enjoy setting up camp near a nice stretch of river

The **Baxter** Bridge State Forest Campground is located on the Manistee River at MI 37 south of Kingsley. Because of the Manistee River, this part of the state is very popular with paddlers of every kind, from solo kayakers and overnight canoeists to large groups of teenaged day-trippers. Depending on where you are on the river, you might see anything from groups on inner tubes to couples paddling inflatable duck boats.

They come here not just because there's nice water for boating but because the land on either side of the river is mostly state and national forest. It's not uncommon to see bald eagles soaring above and river otters playing on the banks. The Manistee also supports an impressive number of fish. Fly-fishing is a big deal up here, but all sorts of anglers come for the bass, walleye, brown trout, and rainbow trout.

Right in the middle of this sits the campground at Baxter Bridge. To be sure, there are other campgrounds, both private and public, on the Manistee, but what recommends Baxter Bridge to the tent camper is that it is not within spitting distance of the popular boat rental spots. The campground is out of the way.

There are two canoe liveries within driving distance of Baxter Bridge—one upriver, one downriver. Neither is less than 12 miles, however, by road. To the east, where the Manistee River passes under US 131, is Chippewa Landing (231-313-0832 or 231-824-3627; chippewalanding.com). Most of the overnight trips they offer begin farther upstream and end at the US 131 bridge. The other outfitter is Wilderness Canoe Trips, located north of Mesick, where the river passes

:: Ratings

BEAUTY: ★ ★ ★ ★
PRIVACY: ★ ★ ★
SPACIOUSNESS: ★ ★ ★ ★ ★
QUIET: ★ ★ ★ ★
SECURITY: ★ ★ ★ ★
CLEANLINESS: ★ ★ ★ ★ ★

:: Key Information

ADDRESS: 6093 East M 115, Cadillac, MI 49601

OPERATED BY: Michigan DNR–Mitchell State Park

CONTACT: 231-775-7911; **tinyurl.com/o3lzspj**

OPEN: Year-round, maintained May–October

SITES: 25

EACH SITE: Picnic table, fire pit

ASSIGNMENT: First come, first served

REGISTRATION: Self-register at campground.

FACILITIES: Hand-pumped water and vault toilets

PARKING: At site

FEE: $13

ELEVATION: 897 feet

RESTRICTIONS:

■ **Pets:** On leash only

■ **Fires:** Fire pits only

■ **Vehicles:** 2 per site; Michigan Recreation Passport required

■ **Other:** 14-day stay limit

under MI 37. The river grows increasingly wider as it flows, and here you can rent canoes, tubes, kayaks, and rafts. They offer customized overnight trips, which give campers a choice between camping primitive on state or federal land, or planning stops at DNR campgrounds like Baxter Bridge.

You don't have to paddle to enjoy Baxter Bridge, though. Many folks just sit next to the river and fish all day. For a bit of an adventure, the campground makes as good a place as any to start a leg on the famed North Country Trail (**northcountrytrail.org**). The trail follows the Manistee River from just west of Tippy Dam Pond, miles to the southwest, and parallels the river upstream to just before US 131. When the trail comes to North 29½ Road (a half mile north of

Baxter Bridge), it leaves the river for a short time, following roads until it can dive back into the state forest.

The campground itself is pleasant. A thick stand of trees serves to divide the campground in half. The first half is in the woods, a small distance from the river. The other half is out in the open. The wooded half of the campground (sites 1–15) has two pit toilets and a hand-pump well, which is located in the area behind site 9. The trees offer a lot of shade, even on the sunniest of days. They also offer more privacy than you will find at the other sites.

The second half of the campground begins as you leave the shade of the woods. Site 16 is on the right, across from the entrance of a small loop of sites closer to the water. Three spacious sites sit out

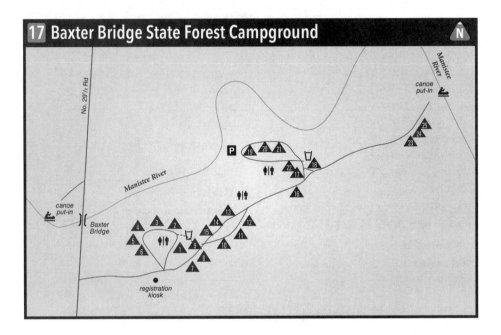

17 Baxter Bridge State Forest Campground

in the sun nearer the main road, but inside the loop are three tightly packed sites. There is a bend in the river here, with access to the water across from site 21 and a small parking area and water access across from site 19. The final three sites, 23–25, are located in an open field just before the canoe put-in. This half of the campground is serviced by a pit toilet and a well close to sites 17 and 18.

:: Getting There

From US 131, take Exit 176 for M 115 west. Continue west for 9.8 miles to South 29 Road, where you will turn right and head north 5.6 miles. The road continues north, changing its name to North 29¼ Road; then comes a sharp turn east and you will find yourself on East 16½ Road. After the route makes another sharp turn, you will find yourself heading north again, this time on North 31 Road. After the next west-north jog, you will see the Manistee River. The campground is east of the road before you get to the bridge.

GPS COORDINATES   N44° 29.508'   W85° 31.632'

18

Arbutus Lake No. 4 State Forest Campground

Almost any day, you can park at the nearby visitor center, walk down to the river, and watch people out for a stroll by the water or sitting in the shade by the banks, with fishing poles in hand.

Traverse City, also known as the Cherry Capital of the World, is at the center of northwest Michigan tourism. And why not? The town rests at the base of Grand Traverse Bay, one of the state's most prized settings. Dozens of hotels, motels, and resorts serve the thousands of visitors who travel to this region for vacation. They come to sit on the beach and play miniature golf. They come for the National Cherry Festival and the Traverse City Film Festival. They come to explore art galleries in nearby Elk Rapids or Suttons Bay. And they come to tour some of the best orchards and wineries in the world.

:: Ratings

BEAUTY: ★ ★ ★ ★
PRIVACY: ★ ★ ★
SPACIOUSNESS: ★ ★ ★ ★
QUIET: ★ ★ ★
SECURITY: ★ ★ ★ ★
CLEANLINESS: ★ ★ ★ ★ ★

Often lost on the casual tourist, however, is the accessibility of nature in and around Traverse City. Few visitors would describe the town as urban in character—a state park is on the main drag, for Pete's sake—but somehow it's easy to miss the trees for the forest.

A few miles southeast of town, where the natural setting is harder to ignore, the state forest maintains the Arbutus Lake No. 4 State Forest Campground on Arbutus Lake. In actuality, five smaller lakes make up Arbutus Lake. All told, they stretch 2 miles from one end to the other, connected by narrow channels. The lakes are numbered, 1 to 5, from south to north. Campers flock to Lake No. 4 throughout the summer, making it one of the state's most popular rustic campgrounds.

This small rustic campground has 25 sites. Campers here come because they love water and woods. The rules for boating on Arbutus Lake favor anglers. A no-wake ordinance on Lakes No. 1 and No. 5 keeps loud water sports to a minimum.

:: Key Information

ADDRESS: 1132 US 31, Traverse City, MI 49686

OPERATED BY: Michigan DNR–Keith J. Charters Traverse City State Park

CONTACT: 231-922-5270; **tinyurl .com/3375tl5.** Canoes can be rented for 4- and 9-mile trips from Ranch Rudolf (231-947-9529; **ranchrudolf .com**), about 6 miles east of Arbutus Lake on Ranch Rudolf Road.

OPEN: Year-round, though snow may prevent access

SITES: 25

EACH SITE: Picnic table and fire pit

ASSIGNMENT: First come, first served; arrive midmorning on the day of stay, and have a plan in place in case the campground is full.

REGISTRATION: Self-register at campground.

FACILITIES: Hand-pumped potable water and pit toilets

PARKING: At site

FEE: $13

ELEVATION: 872 feet

RESTRICTIONS:

■ **Pets:** On leash only

■ **Fires:** Fire pits only

■ **Alcohol:** Permitted

■ **Vehicles:** Michigan Recreation Passport required

And quiet hours are enforced on Nos. 2, 3, and 4. So from 10 at night until 6:30 the next morning, motorboats have to keep to a low speed, and water-skiing is prohibited. Tent campers see this as a boon, especially those who appreciate the sounds of nature when settling into a sleeping bag.

The hilly terrain is a remnant of the last ice age. (As the final glaciers retreated, they left tons upon tons of stones and dirt, scraped up over the centuries of their slow advance.) Camp planners plotted these sites around a steep hill overlooking the north end of Lake No. 4, taking full advantage of the topography. Several of the sites closest to the lake sit above the road or below, requiring campers to park their vehicles alongside the road and take the stairs. Both options provide campsites that overlook the water and keep the road out of sight.

With 25 sites, even when full (that is, every weekend in the summer), the campground remains quiet. Each site has a fire pit and a picnic table. Pit toilets keep with the rustic theme, and campers hand-pump water from the well. In 2009, one of the wells failed, and budget concerns prevented the Forest Service from digging a new one. As a result, the number of campsites had to be reduced, and the campground is actually quieter than it was just a few years ago.

While no readily accessible trails for hiking connect to the campground, the dirt roads in the area wind in and around a dozen or so smaller lakes. These would be fun to explore on a mountain bike. The Arbutus Lake No. 5 Park, operated by East Bay Township, has a beach and nice shady picnic area. The lake itself attracts anglers looking for largemouth bass, and a boat ramp is available. The nearby Boardman River makes for a gentle canoe ride (see left for rental information).

An impressive abundance of wildlife thrives around Arbutus. Visitors often spot blue herons wading in the shallows, and the Michigan Department of Natural Resources designated the entire Arbutus Lake a loon habitat. More than a few bald eagles call the area home, though sightings are still rare enough to be breathtaking. Bald eagles have made a comeback in Michigan, especially in the north. The state now counts nearly 500, from fewer than 100 nests 40 years ago. In fact, authorities removed the birds from the state and federal endangered species lists in 2009.

Though it takes only 10 minutes to drive to Traverse City from the campground, a more ancient waterway connects the two points. The Boardman River flows from headwaters east of Kalkaska. On its way, a nest of lakes southeast of Traverse City indirectly feeds the river—the largest are Spider Lake, Rennie Lake, and Arbutus Lake. Here, pine trees paint the air with their rich scent. The river continues on.

Trace the river on a map and it flows through Brown Bridge (before it was drained), Keystone, and Sabin ponds, and downstream to Boardman Lake. The Boardman River winds through the heart of town to where it empties into the bay. Behind Front Street, tall shady trees line the river. Almost any day, you can park at the nearby visitor center, walk down to the river, and watch people out for a stroll by the water or sitting in the shade by the banks, with fishing poles in hand.

In fact, parks and nature preserves hang on the winding strand of the Boardman like beads on a necklace. Campers looking to stretch their legs and explore will find plenty of fun near the water, from quiet nature hikes to dining in town.

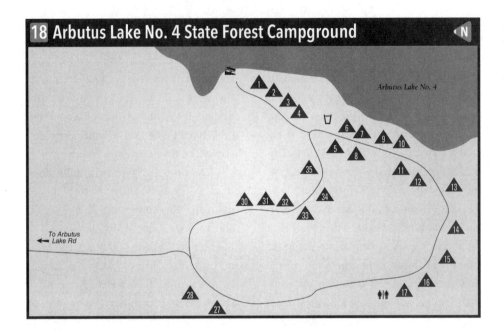

:: Getting There

From US 31, drive 9.5 miles south on Garfield Avenue (which becomes Garfield Road) and turn east on Potter Road (watch for the blinking caution light). Drive a little more than 4 miles to Four Mile Road and turn south. Turn east again on North Arbutus Lake Road, just a half mile on. The park is just less than a mile down on the south side of the road.

Please note: If you are trying another route, maps of the area show Four Mile Road going all the way through to North Arbutus Lake Road from US 31. Not true. It's best to stick with Three Mile Road or Garfield Road.

GPS COORDINATES   N44° 40.716'   W85° 31.350'

19

Bassett Island Campground

This really is the best place to camp if you want to be right on Grand Traverse Bay.

Driving nearly anywhere along the west arm of Grand Traverse Bay, you will recognize the landmark woody dome of Power Island. Not so much its conjoined sibling, Bassett Island, where you will find some of the region's best campsites. The story of Bassett Island cannot be told without reference to its neighbor to the south. A short, narrow causeway that threatens to disappear in years of high water connects Bassett Island's meager 2 acres to Power Island's 202-acre forested mass. On Google maps, the smaller island can be seen only by satellite—the actual map denies its existence altogether. This makes sense, of course. Power Island is a popular Grand Traverse County park. Visitors come by the boatload for the island's beach and exceptional picnic

area. Others anchor their crafts a little ways out from the swimming area, lay out blankets on sunny decks, and do a fine imitation of their sunbathing counterparts on land.

Power Island has gone by many names over the years. Before 1881, the official name was Hog Island. The state legislature changed the name to Marion Island when it was attached to Peninsula Township. Locals still call it Marion Island, as do old guidebooks and numerous maps. At one point, the island was purchased by Henry Ford, and he reportedly camped here with Harvey Firestone and Thomas Edison. During those years, folks called it Ford Island. The island's most recent owners, Eugene and Sadye Power, gave the property over to the county, and it is for them that it is named today.

Bassett Island, however, got its name long ago in the late 19th century from a Civil War veteran, Dick Bassett, who built a cabin here and lived a relatively self-reliant life out on the bay. Later, a steamship company built a dance pavilion on the island. Neither Bassett's cabin nor the dance hall remains. Instead, the county

:: Ratings

BEAUTY: ★ ★ ★ ★ ★
PRIVACY: ★ ★ ★ ★ ★
SPACIOUSNESS: ★ ★ ★ ★
QUIET: ★ ★ ★ ★ ★
SECURITY: ★ ★ ★ ★ ★
CLEANLINESS: ★ ★ ★ ★ ★

:: Key Information

ADDRESS: 1213 West Civic Center Drive, Traverse City, MI 49686

OPERATED BY: Grand Traverse Bay County Parks

CONTACT: 231-922-4818; tinyurl.com/39vvztg

OPEN: Mid-May–mid-October

SITES: 5 (but they can only book 4 at a time)

EACH SITE: Picnic table, grill, fire pit, and raccoon pole

ASSIGNMENT: Call ahead for reservations.

REGISTRATION: Register with ranger on Power Island, or self-register.

FACILITIES: Campground has pit toilet; water on Power Island.

PARKING: At boat launch

FEE: Non-county residents $42; county residents $21 (Sunday–Thursday), $31.50 (Friday–Saturday)

ELEVATION: 579 feet

RESTRICTIONS:

■ **Pets:** On leash only (maximum 6 feet)

■ **Fires:** Fire pits only

maintains five rustic campsites, set apart from the busy day park next door. This really is the best place to camp if you want to be right on Grand Traverse Bay.

Each site has a picnic table, cooking grill, and fire pit. A privy is on the western side of the island, but campers have to purify their own water or carry it over from the well on Power Island. Sites are also equipped with raccoon poles, apparently designed to keep mischievous nighttime prowlers out of your food. That's where the amenities end—at least those provided by the county. Plenty of trees protect sites from wind and sun, and the island's location keeps wandering beachcombers at bay.

During the summer, a ranger and his family live on Power Island. You will

want to call the county park service in advance to reserve a site, but when you get to Power Island, you will register with the ranger or leave payment at the registration station.

Getting to the island is part of the fun. The easiest way is by boat—the 2-mile swim is not recommended for everyone, and it's especially hard with a backpack full of camping gear. Kayakers typically put in at the northern end of Bowers Harbor. The boat launch is just north of the Boathouse Restaurant on Neah-ta-wanta Road. Some paddlers head directly for the island, 2.5 miles away. Others paddle west to Tucker Point, staying within the shelter of Bower Harbor before crossing over to the island—this makes for paddling less open water.

Local outfitters rent kayaks, if you don't have your own (try McLain Cycle & Fitness in Traverse City, 231-941-8855, for weekend or weekly rentals), and many shops lead kayaking trips to the island, teaching novice paddlers the ropes along the way. These instructional trips, however, are usually a round-trip, which is not helpful if you are planning on staying overnight.

Power Island has a number of trails that get little use from the crowds that fill the island's picnic areas. Be sure, also, to leave room in your itinerary for exploring Old Mission Peninsula. From a point just east of downtown Traverse City, the peninsula extends north by northeast into the lower half of Grand Traverse Bay, neatly creating the East Bay and the West Bay. Hiking trails are on the northern end of the peninsula at the Old Mission Lighthouse Park, and the area's gentle hills are popular with cyclists.

Grapes grow well on the peninsula, and a number of wineries take the region's exceptional grape-growing potential and turn it into delicious rieslings and pinots. Summer visitors cruise the scenic Peninsula Drive, visit the Old Mission Lighthouse, and take in a meal at the Boathouse Restaurant or Old Mission Tavern.

For a great view of the West Bay and Power Island, follow Peninsula Drive from Center Road. A little north of halfway up Old Mission Peninsula, Power Island can be seen off to the west, a green hump rising from the water just outside Bowers Harbor. It's an impressive view, prompting more than a few tourists along the way to steer to the side of the road for photographs.

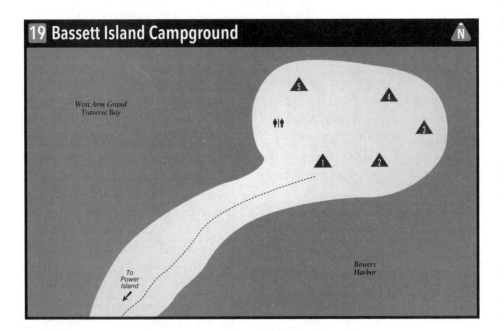

:: Getting There

From US 31 in Traverse City, turn north on M 37 at the base of Old Mission Peninsula. Just about 10 miles along M 37 (also called Center Road), the road veers to the right—stay straight (a left turn) onto 7 Hills Road. In 0.5 mile, turn left on Bowers Harbor Road. Just after you cross Peninsula Drive, the boat launch into Bowers Harbor is on the left. From there, paddle or motor out to the island.

GPS COORDINATES   N44° 52.350'   W85° 34.206'

20

Sleeping Bear Dunes National Lakeshore:

D. H. DAY CAMPGROUND

Campers and day-users come to this sheltered beach for the great view—Sleeping Bear Dunes to the west and Pyramid Point to the east, bookending Lake Michigan and the Manitou Islands.

At the base of the Leelanau Peninsula, you will find one of the state's most dramatic features, Sleeping Bear Dunes, rising nearly 460 feet above Lake Michigan. North of Empire, the South Dune Highway winds through rolling hills and woods thick with maples, beeches, basswoods, and pines. Small inland lakes dot the map, and it is a great drive in the fall when colors are at their peak.

Nestled in the heart of this area, the Sleeping Bear Dunes National Lakeshore's D. H. Day Campground is easily accessible from the short road that

:: Ratings

BEAUTY: ★ ★ ★ ★ ★
PRIVACY: ★ ★ ★ ★
SPACIOUSNESS: ★ ★ ★ ★ ★
QUIET: ★ ★ ★ ★
SECURITY: ★ ★ ★ ★
CLEANLINESS: ★ ★ ★ ★ ★

connects the thriving tourist town of Glen Arbor and the restored historical village of Glen Haven. The state government established the campground as a state park in 1920. Day not only donated the property, but he also chaired Michigan's State Park Commission.

Because the campground is part of the Sleeping Bear Dunes National Lakeshore, the National Park Service maintains the sites. In fact, the NPS maintains two campgrounds here. Of the two, Platte River to the south attracts more campers. It is larger, with paved roads and modern facilities. D. H. Day's rustic facilities—a dirt road, pit toilets, and hand-pumped well water—are not enough, however, to keep the crowds away in the summer.

The campground lies along the shore of Lake Michigan's Sleeping Bear Bay. A path at one end leads to the wide sandy beach. Campers and day-users come to this sheltered beach for the great

:: Key Information

ADDRESS: 8000 West Harbor Highway, Glen Arbor, MI 49636

OPERATED BY: Sleeping Bear Dunes National Lakeshore

CONTACT: 231-334-4634; nps.gov/slbe

OPEN: Early May–late November

SITES: 88

EACH SITE: Picnic table and fire pit

ASSIGNMENT: First come, first served; arrive early morning on the day of stay, and have a plan in place in case the campground is full.

REGISTRATION: Pay at campground office or at its automated pay station (it accepts cash and credit cards).

FACILITIES: Hand-pumped potable water and pit toilets

PARKING: At site

FEE: $12 for camping; a $10 vehicle permit (good for 7 days) is also required for campers and noncamping visitors.

ELEVATION: 596 feet

RESTRICTIONS:

- **Pets:** On leash only
- **Fires:** Fire pits only
- **Other:** Quiet hours 10 p.m.–6 a.m.; camping only on tent pads

view—Sleeping Bear Dunes to the west and Pyramid Point to the east, bookending Lake Michigan and the Manitou Islands.

Campers will find relatively level ground at every site. And though the sites are not as private as some might prefer, they have plenty of room for you to stretch out and enough trees to offer the illusion of seclusion. Generator use is limited to sites 1–31 (for limited hours), so tent campers can enjoy the quiet throughout the remainder of the campground. Group camping is available about a mile away off of M 109 (really a different campground altogether).

Off the main loop, and slightly elevated, sites 57–61 sit a short walk from the water and far from the flow of traffic. Day visitors and campers with an extra vehicle

park in a designated overflow parking area next to site 57, but it still seems nicely set apart.

A combination of sand and prevailing westerly winds formed the dunes a couple thousand years ago. The tallest dunes here are "perched" on the top of limestone plateaus (geologists call this type of dune a perched dune). Like many natural wonders, the forces that created Sleeping Bear cannot be tamed. The dunes here continue to migrate, and significant changes happen over decades and centuries, not millennia and eons.

The federal government established the Sleeping Bear Dunes National Lakeshore, a 72,000-acre national park stretching along 35 miles of Lake Michigan, in 1970. The park incorporates two campgrounds on the mainland and three truly rustic sites on South Manitou Island (also highlighted in this book; see page 87). Backcountry campers can pitch a tent throughout the park and on North Manitou Island, with a permit.

A trip to Sleeping Bear Dunes begins at the visitor center in Empire (at the intersection of M 22 and M 72). There you can learn about the park's numerous hiking trails, the Dune Climb, and the Pierce Stocking Scenic Drive. Built by Pierce Stocking, before the park was even a park, this 7.5-mile loop has numerous overlooks, with views inland toward the picturesque D. H. Day farm and Glen Lake, as well as a short hike to stand 450 breathtaking feet over Lake Michigan.

At the visitor center, you can purchase the vehicle permit necessary for touring the park (and camping), and they can give you directions to the D. H. Day Campground, the northern counterpart to the larger, more modern Platte River Campground.

David Henry Day, the park's namesake, was a relative latecomer to the Sleeping Bear region of Michigan. When he arrived in 1878, the towns of Glen Haven and Glen Arbor were already here.

The lumber industry brought cordwood, which steamships used to power their engines, making Glen Haven one of the busiest stops on the Great Lakes.

Day arrived as the supply of lumber was in decline. With astute foresight, he developed other businesses, buying up portions of Glen Haven in the process. He ran the general store and built the cannery nearby that has served as a fruit processing plant, a warehouse, and now a boat museum. He also bought up vast acreage, much of which he later donated to the state.

In the summer, especially for weekend stays, campers line up in the morning for one of the first-come, first-serve sites. Partly because of this, I enjoy visiting after Labor Day. If you enjoy fall camping, the park can seem nearly abandoned this time of year, and it makes a great base camp for exploring fall colors here and farther north into the Leelanau Peninsula.

Several excellent trails can be found at Sleeping Bear. Many climb the dunes that offer spectacular views. One of the most popular, the Dunes Trail, begins just up the road at the Dune Climb and continues about 1.5 miles out to a view of Lake Michigan.

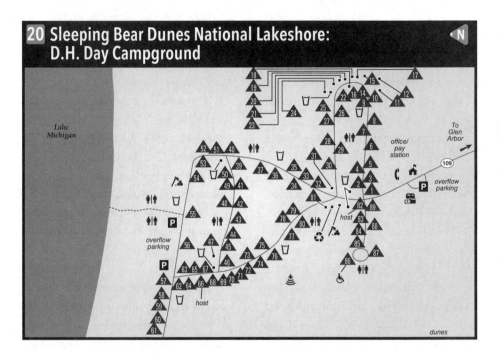

:: Getting There

From points farther south, take US 131 north to M 113. Follow M 37 to Traverse City. From there, drive west on M 72. This road ends at the intersection with M 22 (you'll see the Sleeping Bear Visitor Center) in Empire. Take M 22 north to Glen Harbor, and turn west on M 109; the park is about a mile down on the north side of the road.

GPS COORDINATES   N44° 53.766'   W86° 01.206'

21

Sleeping Bear Dunes National Lakeshore:

SOUTH MANITOU ISLAND, WEATHER STATION CAMPGROUND

The campground faces south with a fantastic view of the Sleeping Bear Dunes across the water.

If **you** visit the historical town of Glen Haven, just west of the D. H. Day Campground in Sleeping Bear Dunes National Lakeshore, you can tour the old Life Saving Service Station, which is now the Coast Guard Station Maritime Museum. The demonstrations here are pretty interesting. They put on a reenactment of the breeches buoy rescue, complete with the firing of the Lyle gun. This complex drill creates a zip line of sorts between a ship that has run aground and the shore, allowing sailors a way to land without jumping into stormy seas. From Glen Haven, the Manitou Islands are clear on the horizon, and the museum does a great job of highlighting the dangers of the Manitou Passage and the lives of the men who tried to make it a bit safer.

People camp on both North and South Manitou Islands. North Manitou is all wilderness, a backpacker's heaven. With the exception of the ranger station, which offers potable water, you're on your own out here. South Manitou, on the other hand, is slightly more developed. Day visitors stay for a few hours and hike a little or take a motorized tour of the island. For overnight guests, the park maintains three rustic campgrounds. Bay Campground is the closest to the ferry dock and ranger station, which are a mile south. Facing east, campers get a view of the Leelanau Peninsula. At the north end of the island, campers walk 3.5 miles from the ranger station to Popple Campground. The site is bare-bones—no potable water, just seven sites, a vault toilet, and (from what I hear) plenty of poison ivy.

:: Ratings

BEAUTY: ★ ★ ★ ★ ★
PRIVACY: ★ ★ ★ ★
SPACIOUSNESS: ★ ★ ★ ★ ★
QUIET: ★ ★ ★ ★ ★
SECURITY: ★ ★ ★ ★ ★
CLEANLINESS: ★ ★ ★ ★ ★

:: Key Information

ADDRESS: 8000 West Harbor Highway, Glen Arbor, MI 49636

OPERATED BY: Sleeping Bear Dunes National Lakeshore

CONTACT: 231-326-5134; nps.gov/slbe

OPEN: Ferry runs early May–mid-October; call ahead at 231-256-9061

SITES: 20

EACH SITE: Shares a community fire pit

ASSIGNMENT: First come, first served

REGISTRATION: Pay for camping and park permit at ferry office.

FACILITIES: Water and pit toilets

PARKING: At the dock in Leland

FEE: $5 for camping; $5/person walk-in fee (in lieu of $10 vehicle permit required elsewhere in the park)

ELEVATION: 599 feet

RESTRICTIONS:

■ **Pets:** Prohibited

■ **Fires:** Fire pits only

The Weather Station Campground lies along the south shore of the island and represents a balance between the other two campgrounds. Farther from the dock but not so rustic as to be uncomfortable, the campground faces south with a fantastic view of the Sleeping Bear Dunes across the water. Prevailing winds here blow from the south, which helps a little during fly season. The sites are tucked in the woods, back from the path. Those along the lake side of the trail have easy access to several paths leading down to the beach. Random groupings of sites share community fire pits.

The island itself has a lot to explore. People have lived on the island for eons. Paleo-Indians hunted here well over 12,000 years ago. More-recent peoples, such as the Ojibwa, camped here as part of their seasonal migrations. The wide, crescent-shaped bay on the island's east edge made

the perfect harbor for ships. And loggers, who were looking for wood to sell to fire steamship engines, found a plentiful supply close to one of the busiest shipping lanes on the Great Lakes. A lighthouse was built to warn ships off the island's shallow point. And soon homesteaders came and tried to make a go of farming.

The ruins of old homesteads, the Island Schoolhouse, several cemeteries, and the lighthouse complex could keep you occupied for a day. A rare stand of white cedars grows in the Valley of the Giants in the island's southwest corner. Some of these trees are more than 500 years old. Why they were spared the lumbermen's saw is a mystery, though some suggest that centuries of sand are embedded in the layers of bark, which would quickly dull any blade and make the task of cutting them down not worth the effort.

Along the west shore of the island lies

a long perched dune—the Bluffs. From atop this sandy mountain, hikers can see the entirety of the island and Lake Michigan all around. It is even said that on the clearest of days, you can see Wisconsin 40 miles to the west. A trail traverses 3 miles of this rise and is well worth the effort. In terms of hiking, many people will hike the beach around the entire island. The trek is all of 14 miles, but it's easy walking. If the water is at a level that allows you to walk on slightly firmer sand, a motivated and energetic hiker can complete the circumference in a day.

Just off the southern shore of the island, not far from the Weather Station Campground, the dangers of the Manitou Passage are clearly illustrated. Visible from the beach, above the water, is the ruined freighter *Francisco Morazan*. It is just one of 16 shipwrecks found in the Manitou Passage Underwater Preserve. Kayakers often paddle out to the rusting hulk for a closer view. And this isn't the only shipwreck you can see from a kayak. *The Three Brothers* off Sandy Point is a 160-foot steamer that sank in 1911. It lies in water 5–45 feet deep.

The Manitou Island Transport ferry out of Leland will take you to and from North and South Manitou Islands. You can take your own vessel, and some have even paddled, but this isn't a trip for the novice. Sudden storms in the passage are legendary—one 19th-century explorer recorded the loss of 50 canoes paddled by Native Americans making the crossing from Sleeping Bear to the islands.

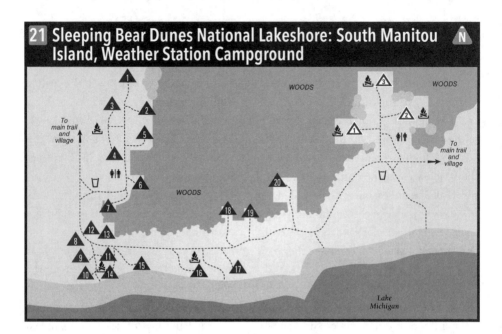

21 Sleeping Bear Dunes National Lakeshore: South Manitou Island, Weather Station Campground

:: Getting There

From Traverse City, take M 22 north to Suttons Bay. Cross west over the Leelanau Peninsula via East Duck Lake Road (M 204). When the road ends, turn north on M 22. In Leland, turn left on River Street. The Manitou Island Transit office is on the dock at the end of Fishtown.

GPS COORDINATES   N45° 00.072'   W86° 06.864'

22

Graves Crossing State Forest Campground

The Jordan was the first waterway in Michigan to be designated a National Wild and Scenic River.

The big territorial surveys of years ago sought to impose some order upon Michigan's wild landscape. In most cases, county and township boundaries line up true—north and south, east and west. County roads follow the same bearings, divvying up the state into manageable grids. We tend to take this superimposed order for granted. It's only when you pay attention to nature that you see things differently. Oddly placed villages and roads that don't line up take on new significance. First, you notice that most towns, for example, are near a lake or river—the bigger the city, the more significant the nearby waterway. When you

see the words portage or traverse on a map, the history of the place suddenly comes to life.

Today, when people only walk cross-country or travel by canoe for recreation, the logic of the old pathways seems part of the dim past. M 66 is a road that defies the usual logic. It sort of staggers north by northwest from Mancelona to East Jordan—getting where it needs to go but always defying a straight line. Stop anywhere along this road and hoof it east into the woods and you will see why. The road is following the curves of the Jordan River. The river springs up from its headwaters northeast of Mancelona and winds south and then north again toward Lake Charlevoix. The lush Jordan River Valley is thick with forest and is a popular destination for fall-color tourists. With steep hills on either side, the upper portion of the river flows through a valley nearly a mile wide.

About 9 miles north of Mancelona, the Mackinaw State Forest keeps a campground at Graves Crossing. Two loops

:: Ratings

BEAUTY: ★ ★ ★ ★ ★
PRIVACY: ★ ★ ★ ★
SPACIOUSNESS: ★ ★ ★ ★ ★
QUIET: ★ ★ ★ ★
SECURITY: ★ ★ ★ ★
CLEANLINESS: ★ ★ ★ ★

:: Key Information

ADDRESS: 2280 Boyne City Road, Boyne City, MI 49712

OPERATED BY: Michigan DNR–Young State Park

CONTACT: 231-582-7523; **tinyurl.com/lya4ff8.** Canoes can be rented on Graves Crossing Road at Swiss Hideaway Canoe Rental (231-536-2341).

OPEN: Year-round, though snow may prevent access

SITES: 10

EACH SITE: Picnic table and fire pit

ASSIGNMENT: First come, first served

REGISTRATION: Self-register at campground.

FACILITIES: Hand-pumped potable water and pit toilets

PARKING: At site

FEE: $13

ELEVATION: 658 feet

RESTRICTIONS:

■ **Pets:** On leash only

■ **Fires:** Fire pits only

■ **Alcohol:** Permitted

■ **Vehicles:** Michigan Recreation Passport required

of five sites each make up the camp. The ground is flat, and the sites are floored with a mix of packed dirt and grass. The woods along this stretch of the river mainly feature pines and cedars, but you will also find the odd maple. Though the river lies just off sites 3, 7, and 8, it keeps its distance. You can hear the river nearby but can only see it through the undergrowth here and there. Both loops share a set of pit toilets and water from a hand pump.

M 66 runs right along one side of the campground. The road is hardly a busy thoroughfare, and there is a wide buffer of trees, but what traffic there is can be heard somewhat in camp. With no host on duty and a short walk from the main road, security is a question. However, as difficult as it is to find the narrow dirt drive into the campground during the

day, I would tend not to worry about troublemakers stumbling in at night.

The Jordan was the first waterway in Michigan to be designated a National Wild and Scenic River. And that it is. The valley here was once logged clean—the lumber was sent down the river to mills in Boyne City and East Jordan. When farmers gave up trying to eke a living out of the poor soil, the state took back much of the land and let it go wild. While it's hard to imagine the ancient forest that was here more than a century ago, the new growth is impressive, especially in the fall when the view from Dead Man's Hill reveals miles upon miles of gold, red, and burnt orange.

Exploring the upper portions of the river means hiking the Jordan Valley Pathway. The lower portion, however, is best explored from the seat of a canoe. Just down the road from Graves Crossing, Swiss Hideaway Canoe Rental rents boats and puts people in the water (see Key Information for phone number). The place can get busy on the weekends. But even with other liveries bringing in groups, the Jordan is hardly an over-paddled river. From the campground to the takeout at Lake Charlevoix is a scenic three- to four-hour float.

For the rest of the river, you will find the main trailhead and parking area for the Jordan River Pathway due east of the campground off US 131 on Dead Man's Hill Road. The quickest way to the trailhead by car takes you 4.2 miles south on M 66 to Alba Road (County Road 620) and then east on Alba Road 4.3 miles to US 131 (also known as Mackinaw Trail). Six miles north you turn left on Dead Man's Hill Road. The trailhead is just 1.7 miles in. The trail closely follows the river all the way back to the Pinney Bridge Campground (Pinney Bridge Road is about 1.5 miles south of Graves Crossing). The trail crosses the road here, but there's no parking area. Access to the campground is limited to those who paddle or hike in. The trail then makes a wide loop south and then north again, crossing many of the creeks that feed the Jordan. It draws close to the river one last time before returning to the trailhead. The entire trip is 18 miles, and many people hike it with backpacks, spending the night at Pinney Bridge.

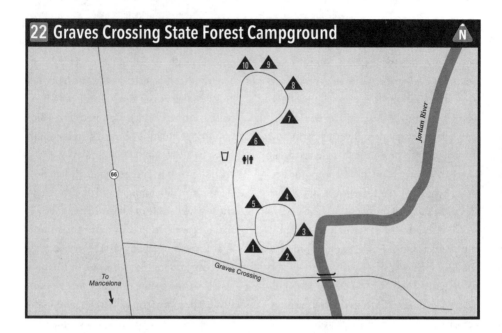

:: Getting There

From Mancelona, head north on US 131/M 66 for 0.8 mile to M 66. Continue north on M 66 for 8.7 miles to Graves Crossing Road. Turn right. The campground is before the bridge on the left.

GPS COORDINATES   N45° 02.016'   W85° 03.918'

Fisherman's Island State Park Campground

The park is truly one of the region's treasures; yet, if it weren't for the small brown signs on US 31, you would miss it altogether.

From **Traverse City** and points south, US 31 parallels the shore of Grand Traverse Bay, about a mile inland. The road essentially shoots straight north from Eastport until you get to the curve into Charlevoix, but the drive is anything but boring. Gently rolling hills make it possible to catch glimpses of Grand Traverse Bay to the west, and orchards, farm markets, and a couple of art galleries line the way. As you approach Charlevoix, the terrain levels out and the road bends to the northeast. Here, between US 31 and Lake Michigan, lies Fisherman's Island State Park.

West of the main road, you find forests of maples, birches, and aspens, as well as cedar bogs and stands of black spruces. Nearly 2,700 acres of secluded forest sit on 6 miles of Lake Michigan shoreline, all surprisingly close to one of the busiest tourist towns in northwestern Michigan. And tucked into this rugged paradise, two surprisingly low-key campgrounds wait on Lake Michigan. The park is truly one of the region's treasures; yet, if it weren't for the small brown signs on US 31, you would miss it altogether.

Much of the history you hear about this stretch of Lake Michigan, between Grand Traverse and Little Traverse Bays, centers on Michigan's lumber heyday. Lumber towns quickly sprang to life along the shore, only to sink back into the wilderness when the lumbermen had cut all they could find and moved on. The long docks of Antrim—immortalized in Nancy Stone's children's novel *Whistle Up the Bay*—used to stretch out into the steel-blue water, just a few miles south of Fisherman's Island State Park. Today, all that is left of Antrim are a cemetery and

:: Ratings

BEAUTY: ★ ★ ★ ★ ★
PRIVACY: ★ ★ ★ ★
SPACIOUSNESS: ★ ★ ★ ★
QUIET: ★ ★ ★ ★ ★
SECURITY: ★ ★ ★ ★
CLEANLINESS: ★ ★ ★ ★ ★

:: Key Information

ADDRESS: Bells Bay Road, Charlevoix, MI 49720

OPERATED BY: Michigan DNR-Young State Park

CONTACT: 231-547-6641; **michigan.gov/fishermansisland**

OPEN: Mid-April–mid-November

SITES: 80

EACH SITE: Picnic table and fire pit

ASSIGNMENT: Reservations can be made online at **midnrreservations.com** and by calling 800-447-2757.

REGISTRATION: Pay campground host at site 1.

FACILITIES: Water and pit toilets

PARKING: At site

FEE: $12 for camping; vehicle permit required (purchase the $10 Recreation Passport when you register your vehicle with the state or at the park; out-of-state visitors pay $8/day or can purchase a pass for $29)

ELEVATION: 642 feet

RESTRICTIONS:

■ **Pets:** On leash only

■ **Fires:** Fire pits only

■ **Alcohol:** Permitted

■ **Vehicles:** Michigan Recreation Passport required

■ **Other:** 15-day stay limit

rumors of submerged posts in the water.

Loggers, however, were not the area's first residents. The Ottawa were living here when Europeans arrived. Earlier still, the Archaic people passed through this way, and archaeologists have found evidence that as far back as 6,000 years ago, the Woodland Native Americans would come here in the summer months to mine the local chert quarries for material to make tools.

Archaeologists left the excavation sites unmarked, but few people come to Fisherman's Island for a history lesson. They come for the woods, the beach, and the excellent camping. A stretch of

private shoreline divides the park into two sections. The northern portion has the campgrounds, marked trails, and picnic areas.

The main road through the north end of the park begins at Bells Bay Road and parallels the shore of Lake Michigan for 2.5 miles. It ends in a gravel parking area at Inwood Creek. Here, you will find a shady picnic area and a narrow footbridge that crosses the creek. Beyond the bridge, a sandy trail continues a couple thousand feet out to a sandy point. The beach can be accessed from anywhere along the path. From here, you can see the island from which the park gets its name. Interestingly, lower water levels have made the island more of a peninsula in recent years.

Loops off the main road define the park's North Campground and South Campground. The North Campground (sites 1–35) has two loops, but campers best appreciate it for a row of sought-after lakeside sites. These campsites (9 and 26–35) are nestled in a band of cedar and birch trees, right on the lake. Just yards from the shore of Lake Michigan, they fill up fast in the summer. The reservation system doesn't allow you to request specific sites at the park. You can, however, note your preference, and they will accommodate the request if a site is available.

The first loop, sites 2–8, is open only to tent camping (site 1 is reserved for the campground host). The sites here have plenty of room to spread out, but there's not much privacy. The second loop of this campground and the South Campground loop, 1.5 miles farther, make good use of the woods. Even campers sited across the road from each other will appreciate a sense of seclusion. The topography gets interesting as you move inland, and the sites on these loops use the steep terrain creatively.

Fisherman's Island Foot Trail, which begins near the park entrance and ends at the parking area at Inwood Creek, offers a pleasant hike that will get you back into the woods. Along the way it follows the ridges behind the two campgrounds. Several trails connect the main path with both campgrounds and the main road. Cross-country skiers and snowshoers use the trail in the winter.

For a more remote adventure, drive south to the southern part of the park. You get there from the village of Norwood. Lake Street, as it is called in town, is a rutted doubletrack that winds 2.3 miles north to Whiskey Creek. Only the most rugged vehicles will make the entire trip. Others will drop to the wayside and their passengers will have to hike the rest of the way.

This section of the park has no amenities—no picnic tables, toilets, or water. As such, visitors have to pack in everything they need. The payoff, however, is nearly 3 miles of unspoiled Lake Michigan beach and access to the remotest parts of the park's sprawling acreage.

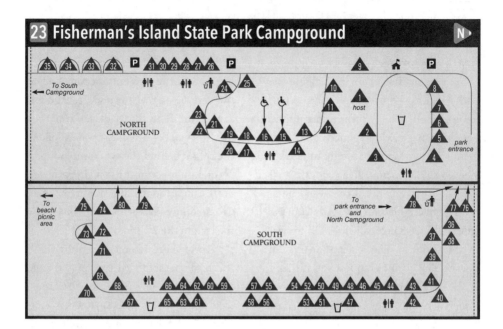

:: Getting There

Bells Bay Road South is right off US 31, about 2.5 miles south of downtown Charlevoix.

GPS COORDINATES   N45° 18.480'   W85° 18.624'

24

St. James Township Campground, Beaver Island

The campground has views of the lake, Garden Island, and nearby Squaw and Whiskey Islands.

During the summer, the ferry out of Charlevoix stays busy carrying passengers (and sometimes their cars, bikes, and kayaks) on the two-hour, 36-mile ride out to America's Emerald Isle, Beaver Island. You can certainly find larger islands in the Great Lakes—seven, in fact, including Manitoulin, Isle Royale, and Drummond Island—but this is the biggest in Lake Michigan and is significantly more accessible than many of its counterparts. Days can be spent riding the island's back roads exploring its two lighthouses, hiking the trails in sections of the Jordan River State Forest, or renting a kayak and paddling along the shore.

:: Ratings

BEAUTY: ★ ★ ★ ★
PRIVACY: ★ ★ ★ ★ ★
SPACIOUSNESS: ★ ★ ★ ★
QUIET: ★ ★ ★ ★ ★
SECURITY: ★ ★ ★ ★ ★
CLEANLINESS: ★ ★ ★ ★ ★

The island, relatively flat with huge swaths of forest, supports two campgrounds—the Bill Wagner Memorial Campground on the east side, just south of Sand Bay, and the St. James Township Campground a half mile west of town on the north side. Both are maintained by the local townships. The Bill Wagner Campground has 22 sites on a wooded lot with views of the northwestern coast of the Lower Peninsula. These sites are rustic, with pit toilets and water from a hand-pumped well.

Closer to town, and much easier to get to from the ferry, the St. James Township Campground has 12 sites, 4 of which have views of the lake, Garden Island, and nearby Squaw and Whiskey Islands. Amenities include a pit toilet and water from a hand pump. Sites at this typical rustic campground sit tucked into the surrounding woods, offering campers privacy. Conveniently, the Emerald Isle Hotel nearby offers campers dedicated showers. For just $10 ($5 for kids), you can clean up from your time of roughing

:: Key Information

ADDRESS: 37735 Michigan Avenue, Beaver Island, MI 49782	**REGISTRATION:** Self-register at campground
OPERATED BY: St. James Township	**FACILITIES:** Hand-pumped well water and pit toilet
CONTACT: 231-448-2505 (chamber of commerce fields questions); **beaverisland.org/camping**	**PARKING:** At site
	FEE: $5
OPEN: Year-round, but not maintained in winter	**ELEVATION:** 612 feet
SITES: 12	**RESTRICTIONS:**
EACH SITE: Fire pit	■ **Fires:** Fire pits only
ASSIGNMENT: First come, first served	

it—soap and towels are part of the deal.

Beaver Island has one of the most fascinating histories you'll find on the Great Lakes. Throughout its history it has been home to various communities. The Ottawa tell of coming to this part of Michigan years back and seeing people who camped and fished from the shores of what they called Turtle Island. The Ottawa themselves never lived on the island. The French named it Île du Castor (or "island of beaver"), the origin of its name today.

In 1844, a seemingly unrelated event would change the island forever. Far south in Illinois, Joseph Smith died, leaving a leadership vacuum at the head of his growing sect, the Mormons. Most of Smith's followers recognized Brigham Young as the true recipient of Smith's mantle, but others followed the charismatic James Jesse Strang. In 1848, Strang moved his church's headquarters to Beaver Island. Soon his followers flooded the island, and Strang declared himself king in 1850. For six years, Beaver Island was home to the only monarchy in U.S. history (though, in all fairness, he only claimed sovereignty over his followers). The Mormons founded the town of St. James, and a small museum is located in the Old Mormon Print Shop in town.

Later, the island was flooded once again, this time by Irish fishermen, most coming from Ireland's County Donegal (hence its nickname, America's Emerald Isle). For a time the island was supplying the most fish coming out of the Great Lakes. Ships stopped here to take on cordwood for fuel or to weather a storm.

From north to south, the island stretches 13 miles; at its widest, it is a mere 6 miles. Excepting times of foul weather, a visitor with a bike has the entire island within an afternoon ride (that is, visitors who don't balk at 26-mile days). Lighthouses are situated at both ends of the island. The St. James Harbor Light directs ships into the island's only safe harbor. At the southern tip of the island, the Beaver Island Lighthouse warns ships that the tricky islands and shallows of the Beaver Island Archipelago lie ahead. The St. James Light is easy enough to find; you will see it from the ferry as you arrive. To get to the southern lighthouse, simply follow East Side or West Side roads south to, you guessed it, South End Road. The lighthouse is open for you to explore. An ornate iron staircase leads to the lantern at the top.

Outside, a steep staircase leads down through the woods to the beach below.

A good part of the southern half of the island falls under the management of the Jordan River State Forest. Part of the forest borders the island's biggest inland lake, Lake Geneserath. This small but deep (50 feet) body of water has a boat launch, and a dozen or so boats are available to rent if you desire to get out on the water. The state forest also has some decent trails for hiking—grab an island recreational trail map at the visitor center for details.

To get to the island, contact the Beaver Island Boat Company (bibco.com) or book a flight with Island Airways or Fresh Air Aviation. Flights are pricier and carry less gear, but they will save you about an hour and 45 minutes of travel time each way.

Kayaks, bikes, and mopeds can be rented at Lakesports & Paradise Bay Gifts in St. James. For supplies, McDonough's Market has a good selection of groceries and other sundries, and the Dalwhinnie Bakery & Deli next door is worth a stop for breakfast or lunch.

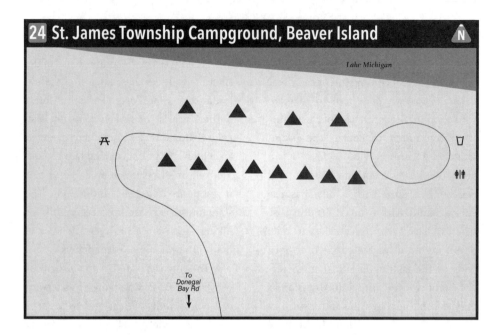

:: Getting There

Take US 31 into downtown Charlevoix and book passage with the Beaver Island Boat Company. The ferry does transport vehicles, for a hefty fee. Cars can be rented on the island cheaply enough at the marina (Geo Trackers). From the dock on Beaver Island, take Main Street south to Donegal Bay Road. The campground is out about 0.5 mile on your right.

GPS COORDINATES   N45° 44.988'   W85° 32.244'

25

Wilderness State Park:

LAKESHORE CAMPGROUND

The cedar trees here are thick, and several tents can sit toward the back of these sites and enjoy privacy lacking elsewhere in the campground.

Just **west** of the Straits of Mackinac, Waugoshance Point juts out into Lake Michigan. The name likely comes from the Potawatomi-Ottawa word for fox—perhaps suffixed with the French word anse for "bay." Interestingly, sailors on the Great Lakes referred to the point as Wobble Shanks. This thin arm of land wraps Sturgeon Bay to the south, and from off the tip of the point, several small, uninhabited islands extend into the passage between the mainland and the Beaver Island Archipelago. This can be a treacherous stretch of water for ships, and those that avoid it tend to follow a path along the northern and western shores of Lake Michigan.

:: Ratings

BEAUTY: ★ ★ ★ ★ ★
PRIVACY: ★ ★ ★
SPACIOUSNESS: ★ ★ ★ ★
QUIET: ★ ★ ★ ★
SECURITY: ★ ★ ★ ★ ★
CLEANLINESS: ★ ★ ★ ★ ★

The Wilderness State Park includes the entire point. All told, the park has 10,512 acres of woods and 26 miles of coastline along Lake Michigan. There are miles of trails for hiking and biking, islands to explore for sea kayakers, excellent beaches for swimming, good fishing for smallmouth bass off the Waugoshance Point, and secluded wilderness cabins on the water for a more sheltered visit.

The park maintains two facilities for camping (well, really one big, divided facility)—the Pines Campground and the Lakeshore Campground. Both are in the vicinity of Big Stone Bay, but the former sits back in pine woods, away from the shore. When recommending a state park to tent campers, there's always some risk. The campgrounds at Wilderness are modern—which translates to flush toilets, water, and electricity (the latter only at some sites). Paved roads run through both camps, and the Pines features paved spurs, a playground, a dining hall, and bunkhouses. The risk is that these places

:: Key Information

ADDRESS: 903 Wilderness Park Drive, Carp Lake, MI 49718

OPERATED BY: Michigan DNR–Wilderness State Park

CONTACT: 231-436-5381; **michigan.gov/wilderness**

OPEN: Early April–November

SITES: 150

EACH SITE: Picnic table and fire pit

ASSIGNMENT: Reservations can be made online at **midnrreservations.com** and by calling 800-447-2757.

REGISTRATION: Register at park office.

FACILITIES: Water and flush toilets

PARKING: At site

FEE: $27 ($16 when the water is off, usually April and October–November)

ELEVATION: 597 feet

RESTRICTIONS:

■ **Pets:** On leash only

■ **Fires:** Fire pits only

■ **Alcohol:** Permitted

■ **Vehicles:** Michigan Recreation Passport required

■ **Other:** 15-day stay limit

are perfect for RVs, motor homes, fifth-wheel trailers, and the like. A state-park official told me that the farther north you go in the state, the fewer of these mobile abodes you typically find in camp. Anecdotally, this appears to be true, but if only one RV pulls into camp with a loud generator and air-conditioning unit and parks next to your tent, it is too many. That said, and with all the risks known, I would recommend pitching your tent at the park's Lakeshore Campground.

Lakeshore sits on Big Stone Bay, overlooking Lake Michigan. The campground has 150 sites, and the beach out front attracts campers from the Pines Campground's other 100 sites. This is the

kind of place where families come for a week. Their children befriend each other on the beach or hang around the vending machine and spend their days walking around in chummy clumps.

The road through camp is essentially one big, flat loop intersected by the road from the camp entrance (essentially making a long crazy-eight). Each half of the campground has modern restrooms (no showers) and drinking water. The individual sites are less uniform here than at the Pines, and campers park their vehicles on gravel-and-packed-dirt spurs. All in all, this lends the campground a more rustic feel than its well-groomed neighbor.

Sites on the inside of the loops back up to each other, and common sense will tell you that the best spots are either those facing the lake or those toward the back of camp against the woods. Of the wooded sites, I think those along the west corner—sites 116, 117, and 120—are the best. The cedar trees here are thick, and several tents can sit toward the back of these sites and enjoy privacy lacking elsewhere in the campground. Those on the water offer the best view, but they come with a price—little cover from the surrounding trees (that is, little privacy), and the beach is the most popular spot in the park, so these sites see more traffic than most. If you come with properly pitched expectations, tent camping at Wilderness can be quite pleasant.

The park itself offers a world of outdoor recreation. With nearly 23 miles of trails to choose from, including a portion of the North Country Trail, hikers can spend days here far from the developed parts of the park. For water sports, sea kayakers will often put in at the end of Park Drive. From here, it's a 3.5-mile round-trip to the tip of the point. West of the point, you will find Temperance Island and Waugoshance Island. Consult a good paddling guide before making this trip. This close to the Straits of Mackinac, you will often see warnings similar to that posted near the campground beach: Paddlers: Beyond the Protection of Big Stone Bay, Currents Dangerous. It is here that Lake Michigan narrows dramatically and flows into Lake Huron.

Historically, the Straits of Mackinac were some of the first places settled by Europeans. Settlements and forts set up at the tip of the mitt and on Mackinac Island and St. Ignace served fur traders and trappers mining the region's abundant wildlife. The state has a cluster of historical state parks in the area to help visitors really experience this aspect of the straits. The closest would be the Colonial Michilimackinac State Historic Park and Old Mackinac Point Lighthouse. Farther afield, you have Mill Creek State Historic Park and Mackinac Island State Park. All of these could take the better part of the day, and they're great fun with kids.

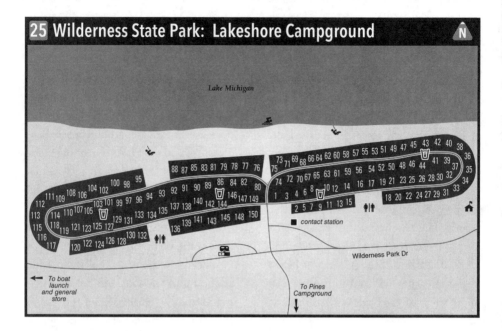

:: Getting There

Take I-75 north to Exit 337, which is Nicolet Street. Turn left at the end of the ramp, driving beneath the I-75 bridge. The first turn is a right on Trails End Road. The road makes a sharp left in 2.5 miles. This puts you on East Wilderness Park Drive. Continue on this road 8.7 miles into the park.

GPS COORDINATES   N45° 44.742'   W84° 53.994'

Northeast Michigan

26

Canoe Harbor State Forest Campground

Access to the South Branch of the Au Sable River makes this campground attractive to paddlers and anglers alike.

Every year during the last full weekend in July, close to 100 canoes take to the Au Sable River in Grayling. Paddlers carry their boats down to the water just before 9 p.m. By the following morning, 14–19 hours later, they cross a finish line in Oscoda, 130 miles downstream. This is the legendary AuSable River Canoe Marathon; since its inception in 1947, it has become one of the country's premier canoe-racing events. As the paddlers prepare for the race, the city of Grayling celebrates with the AuSable River Festival—featuring arts and crafts, pancake breakfasts, and fun runs. And the morning after the paddlers hit the water, a mass of cyclists takes off from town, trying to beat the paddlers to the finish.

:: Ratings

BEAUTY: ★ ★ ★ ★
PRIVACY: ★ ★ ★
SPACIOUSNESS: ★ ★ ★ ★
QUIET: ★ ★ ★ ★
SECURITY: ★ ★ ★ ★ ★
CLEANLINESS: ★ ★ ★ ★ ★

All this takes place during one week in July. The rest of the year, Grayling and the Au Sable River still draw paddlers and tubers (and anglers) from all over. Most of these visitors take a more leisurely approach to enjoying the water. Whether it involves spending the day lying back on an inner tube, going with the flow, or waking before sunrise to claim a choice stretch of water for laying out a hand-tied fly, camping on the river offers a more intimate experience of the Au Sable.

This grand event is missed by the campers at the Canoe Harbor State Forest Campground. The campground is located a half dozen miles south of the Au Sable on the river's South Branch. The main branch has its share of campgrounds, many popular with canoe liveries as places to drop off or pick up clients. The boat launches on the Au Sable see a lot of traffic on summer weekends.

Canoe Harbor has its share of traffic, but it is a quieter alternative. There are group campsites for campers who arrive by canoe, but drive-in visitors have their pick of 44 spacious sites. Each has a fire pit and

:: Key Information

ADDRESS: 11747 North Higgins Lake Drive, Roscommon, MI 48653

OPERATED BY: North Higgins Lake State Park

CONTACT: 989-821-6125; tinyurl.com/k8e46k2

OPEN: Year-round, though not plowed in winter

SITES: 44 (plus 10 canoe group sites)

EACH SITE: Picnic table and fire pit

ASSIGNMENT: First come, first served

REGISTRATION: Self-register at campground

FACILITIES: Hand-pumped water and vault toilets

PARKING: At site

FEE: $13

ELEVATION: 1,128 feet

RESTRICTIONS:

■ **Pets:** On leash only

■ **Fires:** Fire pits only

■ **Alcohol:** Permitted

■ **Vehicles:** 2 per site; Michigan Recreation Passport required

picnic table. Tall pines and mixed hardwoods provide shade for most of the sites.

Folks without a boat or rod might be interested to note that the Mason Tract Pathway passes through the campground. From the trailhead near M 72, the trail meanders 9.6 miles to Chase Bridge Road. It more or less charts a parallel path to the river. The trail makes a short loop around the campground, if you're just looking for an easy way to get down to the water.

On the off chance that the campground is full, you can always check the campgrounds on the Au Sable proper. Burton's Field and Keystone Landing state-forest campgrounds are a short drive (or paddle) away, on the south side of the river. If these are full, which seems unlikely unless you've come up during the canoe

marathon, drive a ways west of Grayling on M 72. The state forest maintains a number of nice campgrounds on the Manistee River. Or you could always follow the Au Sable east. From Grayling to Lake Erie, the river hosts quite a few campgrounds operated by the Au Sable State Forest and the Huron National Forest.

The Au Sable River is certainly an iconic Michigan river, excellent for paddling and fishing. Upstream from Grayling (a town named for a type of salmon that used to thrive, but is no longer found, in the Au Sable), the river sees fewer canoes. Paddling is more a wrestling match in this narrower, shallower, and overgrown portion of the river, though some will rise to the challenge. From Grayling and on downstream, the river swarms with paddlers, tubers, and anglers (especially during summer weekends). Fly-fishermen, in particular, hold the stretch of water from Burton's Landing to the Wakely Bridge in high regard. Nearly 9 miles of the river, known simply as the Holy Waters, are set aside for fly-fishing, with a strict catch-and-release policy. The river here is wide and wadable. It hasn't needed to be stocked in years and naturally supports a strong fishery of trout—mostly brown and brook trout, with a decent population of rainbow.

Downstream, the 23 miles from Mio to the Alcona Dam Pond are designated as the Au Sable National Wild and Scenic River. Established as such in 1984, this section of river has some of the best brown-trout fishing in the Midwest, and paddlers count it among the country's best canoeing.

The closest town, of course, is Grayling. Just north of where US 127 merges with I-75, tourists from the central and eastern parts of the state pass through Grayling and support a strip of fast-food joints and some decent mom-and-pop restaurants downtown. The local economy depends in large part on these travelers, but the military also contributes considerably. Camp Grayling, the largest National Guard training center in the country, takes up huge tracts of land southwest and northeast of town. More than 20,000 people come here for training each year. The rules for exploring land on the Camp Grayling Military Reservation are different from those for the state forest, so if you find yourself roaming off the beaten path, keep an eye out for signs.

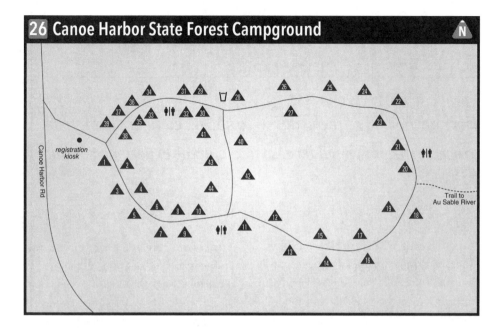

:: Getting There

Exit I-75 for Grayling at Exit 254. Continue north 0.6 mile. Before you come to downtown Grayling, turn right onto M 72. Continue 12.5 miles to Canoe Harbor Road and turn right. The campground is less than a mile down on your left.

GPS COORDINATES   N44° 36.401'   W84° 28.173'

27

Rifle River State Recreation Area: SPRUCE CAMPGROUND

Here at the end of the road, so to speak, campers get a true sense of the park's wilderness and a great experience of the Rifle River.

In the northern half of the Lower Peninsula, few rivers can live up to the reputation of the Au Sable. The river is celebrated for its beauty as much as its recreational value. This close to the Au Sable, you can see why it's easy to miss another of Michigan's great waterways, the Rifle River. The watershed boundary of these two rivers traces a meandering path through northern Ogemaw County. Once used as a shortcut for running lumber down to mills on Saginaw Bay, the Rifle has become a destination river in its own right.

The river pours out of the lakes and streams of the Rifle River State Recreation Area. From there, it flows 47 miles south and east to the bay. Not as grand as its illustrious neighbor, the Rifle offers days of easy paddling and a strong fishery of brown trout and steelhead—perfect for an early morning of fly-fishing or a lazy afternoon float. The nearby campgrounds of the recreation area offer a great base camp for exploring the upper portions of the river or any of the region's other recreational activities—hiking and biking park trails, fishing in nearby lakes and rivers, or relaxing in camp by the water.

The recreation area has four campgrounds. As you drive in from the park entrance at its north end, Spruce Campground is the farthest south, nearly 3.5 miles into the park. Nestled in dense woods on the Rifle River, the campground's 16 sites are plotted around a small double loop, sort of a lazy-eight shape. Few sites at Spruce have room enough for a fifth-wheel. In fact, some sites are cozy enough that only the most humble of pop-ups could squeeze in

:: Ratings

BEAUTY: ★ ★ ★ ★ ★
PRIVACY: ★ ★ ★ ★ ★
SPACIOUSNESS: ★ ★ ★ ★ ★
QUIET: ★ ★ ★ ★ ★
SECURITY: ★ ★ ★ ★ ★
CLEANLINESS: ★ ★ ★ ★ ★

:: Key Information

ADDRESS: 2550 East Rose City Road, Lupton, MI 48635

OPERATED BY: Michigan DNR–Rifle River State Recreation Area

CONTACT: 989-473-2258; **michigan.gov/rifleriver**

OPEN: Mid-April–November

SITES: 16

EACH SITE: Picnic table and fire pit

ASSIGNMENT: Reservations can be made online at **midnrreservations.com** and by calling 800-447-2757.

REGISTRATION: Register at park office.

FACILITIES: Hand-pumped water and vault toilets

PARKING: At site

FEE: $12

ELEVATION: 868 feet

RESTRICTIONS:

■ **Pets:** On leash only

■ **Fires:** Fire pits or in waist-high stoves in the picnic area only

■ **Alcohol:** Permitted

■ **Vehicles:** Michigan Recreation Passport required

■ **Other:** 15-day stay limit

alongside the fire pit. Sites 169 and 172 get you closest to the river, but none are far from the water's edge. Here at the end of the road, so to speak, campers get a true sense of the park's wilderness and a great experience of the Rifle River.

The campground often fills up on the weekends, so plan ahead and make reservations online. If Spruce is full, however, consider one of the park's other campgrounds. Driving into the park, the first you come to is the largest of the pack, Grousehaven Lake. Seventy-five sites, divided into two separate loops, have electric hookups and share modern facilities. Tent campers who appreciate a little luxury should take note of the bathrooms and hot showers at Grousehaven. This is one of the few state parks that keep a modern campground open year-round, and that means heated restrooms in the winter. This is good to know after you've taken an unfortunate dunk in a spring-swollen river, or if you simply want to warm up during colder months.

Assuming you've not come to rent a cabin or camp as a large group, there are just two other campgrounds at Rifle River State Recreation Area, both rustic. The Devoe Lake Campground has 58 sites on Devoe and Jewett Lakes. Divvied up into seven loops, the campground is rather intimate and doesn't feel as big as it really is.

A half mile farther down the way, 25 sites on the Rifle River make up the Ranch Campground. The sites here are large enough for fifth-wheel trailers, and a few trees offer shade. That said, bushes and brush between sites act as a screen between neighbors. Nearby, an open field provides plenty of room for throwing a Frisbee or enjoying a sunny picnic, and a footbridge crosses over the Rifle, carrying hikers to the western edge of the park.

Many campers come this way for the fishing. In addition to the Rifle River, which is popular with fly-fishermen and those who like to cast a line off the bridge near the Ranch Campground, the park has a couple of deep lakes, several shallower lakes, and miles of creek to explore. Devoe and Grousehaven Lakes are both more than 50 feet deep. The other ponds and lakes are less than 20 feet. The most popular with boaters, Grousehaven Lake has a decent fishery of perch, rainbow trout, sunfish, and bass.

It is a shame that many visitors to the recreation area will simply stay close to camp or stake out a lake for fishing and not venture much deeper. The park offers a stellar multiuse trail. A particular favorite with hikers and bikers, the Rifle River Trail winds through 14 miles of the park's interior, following the river for a time and tracing the shore of most of the park's lakes. Mountain bikers will find that most of the pedaling is easy, but the north section of the trail offers some technical challenges.

Many paddlers use the recreation area as a base camp for excursions downstream. Closer to the park and the river's headwaters, the water is shallow and the bank can be overgrown, so most folks put in the Rifle River at Sage Lake Road at the south boundary of the park.

Along the way, the water is smooth and slow and poses little challenge to even novice paddlers. Though they can't really be seen (or readily recognized) from the water, two important archaeological sites lie along the banks of the upper Rifle River. On maps, they are labeled "aboriginal earthworks" and can be found just south of Peters and Selkirk Roads.

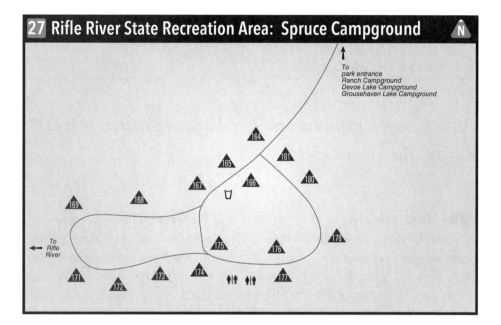

:: Getting There

Take I-75 to Exit 202 (M 33). Continue north on M 33 for 20 miles into Rose City, and then turn right on Main Street. The road changes its name to East Rose City Road. Continue east 4.7 miles until you see the sign for the park entrance on the south side of the road.

GPS COORDINATES   N44° 23.286'   W84° 02.22'

28

Sawmill Point Primitive Campsites

Paths from the individual sites lead down to narrow ledges of earth at the water's edge.

The **Mio Dam** marks a significant change in the Au Sable River. Upstream the watercourse runs unregulated. The Mio Dam, however, widens the river and slows its pace, creating Mio Pond. This dam is the first portage on the Au Sable, and the four dams and four flood ponds that follow create a river that is a far cry from the one paddled by Native Americans and early European explorers, or even the loggers who used the river to float their lumber to Lake Huron. Much of this stretch of the Au Sable lies within the Huron National Forest, and the U.S. Forest Service has made good use of the recreational opportunities these dams create.

:: Ratings

BEAUTY: ★ ★ ★ ★ ★
PRIVACY: ★ ★ ★ ★
SPACIOUSNESS: ★ ★ ★ ★
QUIET: ★ ★ ★ ★ ★
SECURITY: ★ ★ ★ ★
CLEANLINESS: ★ ★ ★

The largest of these man-made lakes is Cooke Pond, and high on a bluff overlooking the pond, you will find the centerpiece of the Huron National Forest— the Lumberman's Monument and Visitor Center. The monument itself is a 14-foot bronze sculpture of three loggers. Erected in 1931, the center was built by the Civilian Conservation Corps, who also planted the large pine trees visitors enjoy today. You may find it ironic that a national-forest monument celebrates the industry that harvested most of the state's forests, but logging was a fact of life in northern Michigan, and this visitor center does a great job of telling that story.

Adjacent to the Lumberman's Monument and Visitor Center, people can set up camp at the Monument Campground. The sites are rustic, and the campground amenities are limited to vault toilets and drinking water. Farther afield, however, a number of primitive sites are available in the form of a dispersed campground. These would be the 42 sites (numbered 32–73) found up and down the length of

:: Key Information

ADDRESS: 5761 North Skeel Avenue, Oscoda, MI 48750

OPERATED BY: Huron-Manistee National Forest Huron Shores Ranger Station

CONTACT: 989-362-8961; **tinyurl.com/n4c29ow**

OPEN: Year-round

SITES: 16

EACH SITE: Fire pit

ASSIGNMENT: Reservations required May 15–September (877-444-6777; **recreation.gov**); first come, first served October–May 14

REGISTRATION: Register and pay for camping permit at Lumberman's Monument and Visitor Center.

FACILITIES: Hand-pumped water and vault toilets

PARKING: At site

FEE: $10/night and $9 one-time reservation fee; no fee October–May 14

ELEVATION: 701 feet

RESTRICTIONS:

■ **Pets:** On leash only

■ **Fires:** Fire pits only

Cooke Pond. These sites vary in accessibility. On the campground map, sites are coded with a C, D, or W for canoe access, drive-in, or walk-in, respectively. For this book, we will be looking at the 16 drive-in sites the U.S. Forest Service calls the Sawmill Point Primitive Campsites. But be aware that 26 more sites await campers looking for a little adventure. For example, Horseshoe Island is a popular scenic feature of Cooke Pond, visible from the overlook at the visitor center. Few of the travelers passing through realize, as they take in the sweep of landscape, that they could camp on that idyllic island. Instead, they snap a few photos, round up the kids, and head off for the next stop. The few in the know, however, reserve the campsite ahead of time, make the 1.5-mile paddle out to campsite 41-C, and enjoy a unique experience of nature.

Sawmill Point offers a similar experience for campers not able to paddle or hoof it to one of the less accessible sites. The point juts out into Cooke Pond a mile or two downriver from the Lumberman's Monument. The terrain here drops sharply to the pond. You can only imagine how much more impressive these bluffs and valleys must have appeared when the water was at its normal levels. Sites are split between the northeast and southwest sides of the point. Sites 48–57 edge the northeast side of the point, all from a single road. Sites 42–47 are on their own loop.

All but two (46 and 47) of the campground's 16 sites overlook the water.

Paths from the individual sites lead down to narrow ledges of earth at the water's edge. It would be hard to lower a canoe to the river from camp, but thankfully the campground has a boat launch. There's an overall shaggy feel to the place, but it's a primitive campground—the vault toilets and hand-pumped water are luxuries—and if you find landscaping important, definitely choose one of the other national-forest campgrounds nearby (Monument and Rollways are always good bets). The campground is popular with anglers and others looking for a base close to the water.

This section of the Au Sable River is on the Lumberman's Monument Auto Tour. This scenic 68-mile drive begins at the Tawas Point State Park and makes a crooked loop up to the monument, over to Oscoda, and back to Tawas. Along the way it passes museums, historical markers, and quite a few natural sites. You can

pick up a brochure at the state park. One stop on the tour you shouldn't miss is Iargo Springs. Just 3 miles west of the monument on Iargo Road, the springs here were once used by Native Americans. During the logging years, lumbermen dammed the springs and diverted the water to their camps. You can follow the water's path toward the river as it flows downhill over a number of man-made dams. It's a 300-step stairway down, so keep in mind that you'll have to walk back up.

While the Au Sable plays a central role in the region's recreational opportunities, there's more here than just paddling. The Highbanks River Trail begins at the main road into Sawmill Point and continues west, following the river. The 6.3-mile route passes the Lumberman's Monument and Canoers Memorial Monument before ending at Iargo Springs. This is a favorite trail with hikers and cross-country skiers.

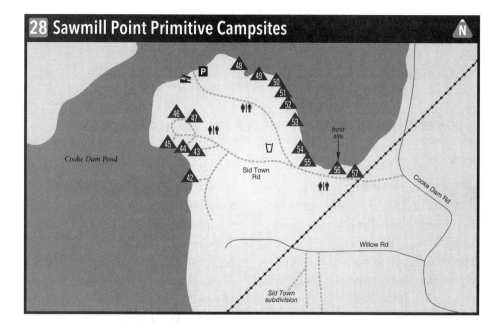

28 Sawmill Point Primitive Campsites

Cooke Dam Pond

Sid Town Rd

host site

Cooke Dam Rd

Willow Rd

Sid Town subdivision

:: Getting There

From US 23 in Oscoda, follow West Mill Road west. It quickly becomes East River Road and then just River Road. Whatever the name, follow the road 14.3 miles. Turn right (north) on Cooke Dam Road. Drive 1.5 miles and turn left on Sid Town Road. You're there.

GPS COORDINATES   N44° 27.342'   W83° 36.366'

29

Ossineke State Forest Campground

If you are looking to leave people behind, this is your spot.

On a beautiful summer day, as clouds lazily float in front of a bright blue sky, their shadows dappling the sandy beach at the southern end of Thunder Bay, it's hard to imagine that you're looking out over one of the most dangerous stretches of water in the Great Lakes. Lake Huron is the second largest of the lakes, and sailors making the turn south from the Straits of Mackinac know that it pays to keep a keen eye on the weather.

Ever since Robert de La Salle began exploring the Great Lakes by sailing ship, wrecking first the *Frontenac* in 1679 and then losing the legendary *Le Griffon* later that year, these freshwater seas have taken thousands of ships, and few spans of water are as treacherous as those off North Point and Thunder Bay Island. To protect the

cultural legacy of these wrecks, the area was designated an underwater preserve by the state in 1981. Nineteen years later, an agreement with the National Oceanic and Atmospheric Administration (NOAA) established the Thunder Bay National Marine Sanctuary—jointly managed by the state and NOAA. So far, more than 200 ships have been found within the boundaries of the preserve.

The Ossineke (pronounced "AH-sin-eek") State Forest Campground, a few miles northwest of South Point, overlooks the southern end of Thunder Bay. Neatly tucked between the small unincorporated village of Ossineke and the water, the park caps off a section of Lake Huron shoreline that's bordered to the south by Mackinaw State Forest, Negwegon State Park, Au Sable State Forest, and Huron National Forest, all in sprawling succession.

From above, the campground looks like an unbalanced mobile. Drive into the park and you come to a T. Turn left to find another T, off of which balances a long road with turnaround loops at each end. Here, you find sites 1–17 and 18–26. If, on

:: Ratings

BEAUTY: ★ ★ ★ ★ ★
PRIVACY: ★ ★ ★ ★
SPACIOUSNESS: ★ ★ ★ ★ ★
QUIET: ★ ★ ★ ★ ★
SECURITY: ★ ★ ★ ★
CLEANLINESS: ★ ★ ★ ★ ★

:: Key Information

ADDRESS: 248 State Park Road, Harrisville, MI 48740

OPERATED BY: Michigan DNR– Harrisville State Park

CONTACT: 989-724-5126; tinyurl.com/2cxjxqe

OPEN: Year-round, though not plowed in winter

SITES: 42

EACH SITE: Picnic table and fire pit

ASSIGNMENT: First come, first served

REGISTRATION: Self-register at campground

FACILITIES: Hand-pumped water and vault toilets

PARKING: At site

FEE: $13

ELEVATION: 577 feet

RESTRICTIONS:

- **Pets:** On leash only
- **Fires:** Fire pits only
- **Vehicles:** Michigan Recreation Passport required

the other hand, you turn right, the main road leads to sites 27–42, with a loop of their own.

Driving in from Ossineke, following the main drive left, you will first notice a pleasant picnic area with a view of the lake. To the left, sites 1–17 alternate from the water side to the wooded side of the drive. Site 9 is reserved for the campground host. Sites 15 and 17, in particular, enjoy a great view of the bay. Unique to site 15 is the grave marker of one A. J. Michalowsky. In 1865, this 26-year-old man drowned while attempting to sail from Ossineke to Alpena. His body washed up here, and here he was buried—another testament, I suppose, to Shipwreck Alley's dangerous reputation.

To the right of the picnic area, far fewer sites sit on the wooded side of the road—most are on the water. At most

sites, stands of pines, cedars, and maples screen the view of the bay, but they also serve to protect campsites from winds off the beach. Here and there, you will find paths cutting through to the water.

This is a great campground for swimming—but keep in mind that the Great Lakes are always a bit chilly. The beach is mostly sandy. The water here is shallow, and if you wear lake shoes for the rocks, you can walk quite a ways out into the bay.

Two islands—Scarecrow and Bird—wait on the horizon, a few miles offshore to the east. Kayakers find it an enjoyable paddle to follow the shore of South Point from the Black River in Negwegon State Park. From there, they launch a mile into the lake to Bird Island and then leapfrog to Scarecrow Island. Between these two lies the closest shipwreck to the campground. The *William H. Stevens* rests in

10 feet of water. This 117-foot schooner sank with a cargo hold full of wheat in the fall of 1863. There was no recorded loss of life with this sinking, so any phantom sailors you see wandering the beach at night are merely the result of an overactive imagination.

The Ossineke State Forest Campground has one hiking trail, the 1-mile Ossineke Pathway, but with so much state- and national-forest land around, hikers will find trails enough for exploring. Just to the south in the Negwegon State Park, there are 11.6 miles of path on three separate trails. The terrain here varies, and paths often pass through boggy swampland, so getting your feet wet is not unlikely.

Negwegon is an undeveloped park, and just getting there is a bit of a feat. The main road to the park entrance is the aptly named Sand Hill Road, and officials warn that a four-wheel-drive vehicle is often the only way to get through the road's sandy patches. Once you're in, the park offers potable water, an outhouse, and four backcountry campsites. If you are looking to leave the world behind, this is your spot.

If you are looking for some civilization, Alpena is 12 miles north on US 23. There, you can learn more about the Thunder Bay National Marine Sanctuary by visiting the Great Lakes Maritime Heritage Center. This maritime museum tells the story of the boats that have gone down near Thunder Bay through detailed exhibits, models of various ships, and a life-size deck that gives visitors the feeling of being aboard a ship in a storm on Lake Huron.

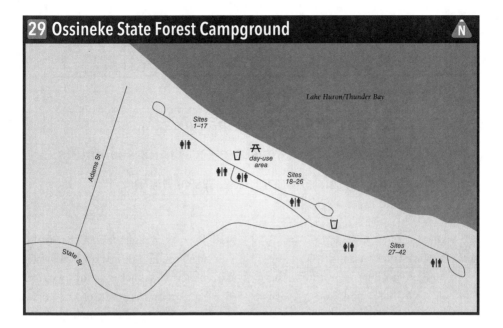

:: Getting There

From US 23 in Ossineke (12 miles south of Alpena), head east on Ossineke Road. In 1 mile, turn right onto State Street. The campground is at the end of the street.

GPS COORDINATES   N44° 27.342'   W83° 36.366'

30

Tomahawk Creek Flooding State Forest Campground

Few places are as enjoyable for camping as this site, surrounded by thick woods, pleasant water for swimming and fishing, and trails enough for days of hiking.

Southeast of Onaway in the Mackinaw State Forest is one of the state's more unique geological features—the Sinkhole Area. The region is dotted with deep wooded sinkholes, small lakes, and a number of nearby rustic state-forest campgrounds, including this one on Tomahawk Creek Flooding. Few places are as enjoyable for camping as this site, surrounded by thick woods, pleasant water for swimming and fishing, and trails enough for days of hiking.

That said, the scenery on the drive in from M 33 can be downright discouraging. The Tomahawk Lake Highway passes through flat terrain lined with grass and scrubby trees. It might be enough to make you turn around, but fear not: the destination more than makes up for the drive. The campground is south of the "highway" off of Dam Road (1 mile in from M 33). Other campgrounds can be found farther along on Shoepac and Tomahawk Lakes. They are both nice spots for camping (though Shoepac seems better suited for fifth-wheel trailers and RVs). On the off chance that both units of the Tomahawk Creek Flooding State Forest Campground are full, campers should find a site at one of these excellent alternatives.

The Tomahawk Creek Flooding is the largest body of water in this section of the Atlanta State Forest. The campground on the north shore of the man-made lake is actually divided into two sections: the West Unit and the East Unit. Here, we look at the 24 sites that make up the West Unit. On the map, nearly half of these are on the water, but, in reality, some have better access than others. Site 22, for example, has a particularly nice view of the lake.

:: Ratings

BEAUTY: ★ ★ ★ ★
PRIVACY: ★ ★ ★
SPACIOUSNESS: ★ ★ ★ ★
QUIET: ★ ★ ★ ★ ★
SECURITY: ★ ★ ★ ★
CLEANLINESS: ★ ★ ★ ★

:: Key Information

ADDRESS: 4347 Third Street, Cheboygan, MI 49721	**FACILITIES:** Hand-pumped water and vault toilets
OPERATED BY: Aloha State Park	**PARKING:** At site
CONTACT: 231-625-2522; tinyurl.com/lkm7ao2	**FEE:** $13
OPEN: Year-round, though not plowed in winter	**ELEVATION:** 856 feet
SITES: 24 (West Unit)	**RESTRICTIONS:**
EACH SITE: Picnic table and fire pit	■ **Pets:** On leash only
ASSIGNMENT: First come, first served	■ **Fires:** Fire pits only
REGISTRATION: Self-register at campground	■ **Alcohol:** Permitted
	■ **Vehicles:** 2 per site; Michigan Recreation Passport required

That said, there's hardly a bad place to pitch a tent here. With spacious, grassy sites and plenty of shade from pines and the usual assortment of hardwoods, the campground sites offer room to spread out and a decent amount of privacy.

(If your campers are more interested in swimming than fishing, however, the campground on Tomahawk Lake might be a better choice. There's a day-use area with a sandy beach, and some of the campsites are close enough to the shore that you could presumably slip straight from the tent into the water.)

The campground has a boat launch, as do Tomahawk Lake, Little Tomahawk Lake, Shoepac Lake, and Francis Lake. There's no end to the fishing holes anglers might find. Fisheries here boast bluegill and largemouth bass. Off-road vehicles are restricted in the campgrounds themselves, but there is an abundance of trails for the off-road enthusiast.

The state forest's most interesting and scenic features are the sinkholes just north of the Tomahawk Lake Highway. Not only does the 2.5-mile loop offer a pleasant nature hike, but it's also a chance to see geological forces in action.

Campers interested in understanding the geology of the Sinkhole Area will first learn a little about karst topography. This is when a layer of bedrock erodes, causing the ground above it to sink. In the case of northern Michigan, the bedrock is limestone and the ground above it is glacial till. (Glacial till is the sediment that the glacier scraped up as it advanced. When it retreated, it left behind piles of this rubble everywhere. The glaciers really defined the landscape here.)

Groundwater seeps down through the till and eats away at the limestone, which dissolves very easily for a rock. When enough limestone is gone, the foundation collapses. Sometimes these depressions hold water and become lakes. Other times all that is left is a conical hole in the ground. The sinkholes are still active. On the eastern edge of Shoepac Lake, you can see collapses that occurred in 1937 and 1976.

Motor vehicles are prohibited in the 2,600 acres that make up the Sinkhole Area. The Sinkhole Pathway makes a wide loop around the area's five most dramatic holes. Observation decks at each sinkhole offer nice views and give you a real sense of the dramatic landscape. There are stairs at the first sinkhole for hikers inclined to make the 181-step trek to the bottom and back.

In 1939, a forest fire swept through this area, destroying nearly 40,000 acres. Along the pathway, you can still see evidence of this fire. The trail also passes through thick stands of aspens and jack pines, which have grown since the fire.

For more adventurous hikers, especially those with a good map and compass, the Sinkhole Area is lined with fire lanes. The map at the trailhead has some of these marked out, but there are more to explore. The parking area and trailhead for the Sinkhole Pathway are just north of the Shoepac Lake State Forest Campground.

Another popular hike passes through the East Unit of the Tomahawk Creek Flooding campground—the 80-mile High Country Pathway, designed to offer backpackers a week of hiking in the wilderness. There is really no other trail like it in the Lower Peninsula. Other campgrounds on the pathway include Pigeon River (see page 128) and nearby Shoepac Lake. For day-hike purposes, the trail connects with the Sinkhole Pathway.

In recent years, mountain bikers have taken on the challenge of the High Country Pathway. The entire 80 miles represents sort of a marathon of mountain biking, and a careful cyclist can complete the loop in one day—usually by riding from sunup to a little after sundown. Considered an epic ride by the International Mountain Biking Association, this course requires that you be well prepared. You certainly don't want to find yourself 40 miles in with a mechanical problem and no backup plan.

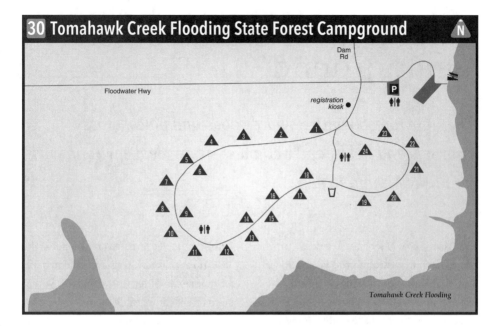

:: Getting There

From Gaylord (Exit 282 on I-75), drive 33 miles east on M 32. In Atlanta, turn north on M 33. In 15.5 miles, turn right on Tomahawk Lake Highway. After 1 mile, turn right on Dam Road. Follow signs for campground.

GPS COORDINATES   N45° 12.784'   W84° 11.099'

31

Pigeon River State Forest Campground

The state forest—with its hardwoods and pines, grassy clearings and fields, and wetlands—is an ideal environment for Rocky Mountain elk.

Three of Michigan's finest trout waters flow through the Pigeon River Country State Forest—the Sturgeon, the Pigeon, and the Black Rivers. In the early part of the last century, Ernest Hemingway made his way often to the Black River and spent days casting a line, nights sleeping under the open sky. In his ever-so-concise style, he called this little piece of country "the pine plains east of Vanderbilt."

In 1919, the "pine plains east of Vanderbilt" were incorporated as a state forest, protecting the last big tract of almost-wild wilderness in the Lower Peninsula. Not quite untouched, Pigeon River Country was logged and left for scrap by lumbermen. Forest fires raged here, the last in 1939. Today, we have 118,000 acres of managed wilderness, complete with a herd of elk comparable to none other this side of the Mississippi.

The state forest has seven rustic campgrounds. Most are on small lakes; one is set aside for equestrian camping. Driving in from Vanderbilt on Sturgeon Valley Road, you pass close by three of them—Pickerel Lake, Pigeon Bridge, and Round Lake. The fourth, however, is the one you want. North on Twin Lakes Road, less than a mile past the Pigeon River Country Field Office, is the Pigeon River State Forest Campground (not to be confused with Pigeon Bridge).

The campground is on a small bend of the Pigeon River. There are 19 campsites, 15 on a main loop. Sites 1–6 (with the exception of 5) sit right on the water. Sites 7–15 complete the loop. The remaining four sites are a bit removed, east of the main road into the campground. Site 19 is particularly attractive. The site is wide

:: Ratings

BEAUTY: ★ ★ ★ ★
PRIVACY: ★ ★ ★ ★ ★
SPACIOUSNESS: ★ ★ ★ ★
QUIET: ★ ★ ★ ★ ★
SECURITY: ★ ★ ★ ★ ★
CLEANLINESS: ★ ★ ★ ★ ★

:: Key Information

ADDRESS: 7136 Old 27 South, Gaylord, MI 49735

OPERATED BY: Michigan DNR-Otsego Lake State Park

CONTACT: 989-732-5485; tinyurl.com/nghl22p

OPEN: Year-round, though not plowed in winter

SITES: 19

EACH SITE: Picnic table and fire pit

ASSIGNMENT: First come, first served

REGISTRATION: Self-register at campground

FACILITIES: Artesian well and vault toilets

PARKING: At site

FEE: $13

ELEVATION: 887 feet

RESTRICTIONS:

■ **Pets:** On leash only (maximum 6 feet)

■ **Fires:** Fire pits only

■ **Vehicles:** 2 per site; Michigan Recreation Passport required

open, right on the water where Ford Lake Road crosses over the Pigeon. There is a notable lack of privacy here, however. There are no trees, it's right on the road, and there's an unobstructed view of the parking area for day visitors.

Sites along the water are more or less grassy. The others are nestled in pine woods, fringed by ash and other hardwoods. These wooded sites are floored with the reddish hue of fallen pine needles.

Water is provided by an ever-flowing artesian well. Two vault toilets are in the middle of the loop. Access is easy enough, unless you're walking over from sites 17–19. It's not terribly far (less than 0.2 mile), just not as convenient.

The 3-mile stretch of the Pigeon River, from Sturgeon Valley Road to the campground, is wide (20–40 feet) and shallow (rarely deeper than 4 feet). This is the first section of the river considered accessible for paddlers—you can paddle a bit upstream, but the river becomes too small and obstructed to enjoy the trip.

Because the water is wide, shallow, and relatively even-bottomed, anglers of all stripes wake early in the morning, don waders, and try their luck catching brown trout and brook trout. Many stay at the campground, though many camp elsewhere and drive in early.

The 80-mile High Country Pathway passes through this campground. Tracing a large loop through portions of Mackinaw and Pigeon River Country state forests, the trail was designed for hikers looking for a week of backpacking. The pathway connects a number of state-forest campgrounds (including Tomahawk Creek Flooding on page 124).

For shorter hikes, the Shingle Mill Pathway offers 6-, 10-, and 11-mile loops. The main trailhead is at Pigeon Bridge, and the trail follows the river for a time. The High Country Pathway connects with a portion of this trail.

In recent years, mountain bikers have secured the right to use the Shingle Mill and High Country pathways. It took some convincing, but the mountain-biking community has developed a reputation for respecting hikers and caring for the trails. In 2006, the International Mountain Biking Association added the High Country Pathway to its list of epics, calling the route a "soul searcher."

A year before the state forest was officially established, seven elk were released into the wild here. The native elk became extinct, so Rocky Mountain elk were introduced in an attempt to restore a viable herd. The state forest—with its hardwoods and pines, grassy clearings and fields, and wetlands—is an ideal environment for these animals.

The elk made themselves at home, and today the herd has more than a thousand.

The elk are most active in September, when the bulls are looking to make a name for themselves in the herd—a lot of bugling and playing rough with the brush. Most nature watchers come out on the weekends, so your best bet is to come during the week. Or better yet, come in late April or early May. There are few crowds in the spring, yet the elk are out feasting on fresh vegetation.

The west part of the wilderness is a 6,300-acre no-motor area called Green Timbers. Hiking and cross-country-skiing trails appeal to some, and hunters make good use of the woods.

In the late 1960s and early 1970s, energy companies began pushing for more access to Pigeon River Country. The presence of oil and gas raised questions about proper land use within a designated wilderness area and led to an extended court battle. In 1979, a Michigan Supreme Court decision led to a compromise allowing for drilling in the southern third of the forest.

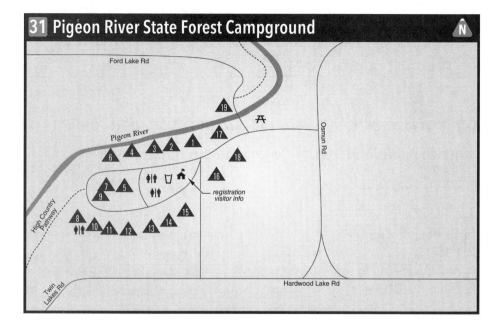

:: Getting There

From I-75 take Exit 290. Head south on Mill Street to the intersection in Vanderbilt (0.5 mile). Head east on East Sturgeon Valley Road. Drive 11.5 miles to Twin Lakes Road. Turn north and drive 1.7 miles to the campground entrance. The field office is about a half mile before the campground.

GPS COORDINATES   N45° 10.596'   W84° 25.668'

32

Ocqueoc Falls State Forest Campground

Close your eyes, dangle your feet in the water, and contemplate the quiet current of geological circumstance that created this place.

North of the Mackinac Bridge, Michigan is a land of waterfalls. From Tahquamenon to Bond, the Upper Peninsula is flush with falling waters. South of Big Mac, however, it's slim pickings. Ocqueoc is the only named waterfall in the Lower Peninsula. (There is one unnamed falls. On a small stream that feeds the Manistee River, it is less accessible and not as picturesque.) The name of the river and falls is pronounced "AH-key-ock," which many say meant "crooked river" to the Ojibwa who lived here. Virgil Vogel, author of *Indian Names in Michigan*, however, says that definition has no basis in the Ojibwa vocabulary. Thus,

according to this expert at least, its meaning remains a mystery.

Here, where the often-twisty Ocqueoc River becomes Ocqueoc Falls, the water is edged by a stone bank. Along the rock's weathered top, you can just make out the shapes of fossilized shells . . . or are they some kind of plant? In either case, with little else but kids playing in the falls and some adults wading upstream, it's easy to close your eyes, dangle your feet in the water, and contemplate the quiet current of geological circumstance that created this place.

The Ocqueoc day-use area and campground sit across the road from each other. Arrayed in a single loop, campsites along the campground's west and southwest edge are on the Ocqueoc River. A bluff raises half of the sites slightly above the others. The campground is what you might expect if you're familiar with camping at state-forest facilities. There are pit toilets, and you can pump drinkable water from the well.

:: Ratings

BEAUTY: ★ ★ ★ ★
PRIVACY: ★ ★ ★ ★
SPACIOUSNESS: ★ ★ ★ ★ ★
QUIET: ★ ★ ★ ★ ★
SECURITY: ★ ★ ★ ★ ★
CLEANLINESS: ★ ★ ★ ★

:: Key Information

ADDRESS: 5001 US 23, Rogers City, MI 49779

OPERATED BY: Michigan DNR–P. H. Hoeft State Park

CONTACT: 989-734-2543; tinyurl.com/2at4kkk

OPEN: Year-round, though not plowed in winter

SITES: 13

EACH SITE: Picnic table and fire pit

ASSIGNMENT: First come, first served

REGISTRATION: Self-register at campground

FACILITIES: Hand-pumped well water and pit toilets

PARKING: At site

FEE: $13

ELEVATION: 706 feet

RESTRICTIONS:

■ **Pets:** On leash only

■ **Fires:** Fire pits only

■ **Vehicles:** 2 per site; Michigan Recreation Passport required

The sites are mostly grassy, with packed dirt and gravel spurs. Shade comes from a mix of maples, oaks, white pines, and beeches. The first couple of sites on the water, 4 and 5, enjoy the least privacy but have the best views of the river. Sites 7–10 sit on the bluff and, with the exception of site 9, directly overlook the water. If privacy is your thing and being on the water isn't a requirement, sites 12 and 13 were custom-made for you. Found at the far side of the loop, these sites are deep, backing into a wood of tall pines—very spacious and set apart from the rest of the campground.

Waterfalls typically indicate a change in geology that often goes unnoticed on dry land—and a lot is going on geologically in this part of the state. The region's karst topography (see also Tomahawk Creek Flooding on page 124) means that layers of bedrock beneath the surface are slowly eroding. Near Tomahawk and Shoepac Lakes, this has resulted in sinkholes. You can also find sinkholes in Alpena County, and even under the waters of Thunder Bay. Near Ocqueoc, it is said that the Little Ocqueoc River, a tributary of the Ocqueoc, flows underground for a portion of its path, and, at one point, one of its branches can be seen flowing out of a hill. The website for the town of Onaway indicates that you can see this for yourself about a mile north of M 68 on Silver Creek Road—this would be just a few miles from the campground, but I've been unable to locate the spot.

But the most fun you can have on the water typically occurs aboveground. Let's begin with the waterfall. The Ocqueoc

River drops 5–6 feet at the falls. Certainly no Niagara, the falls are tall enough to be interesting yet short enough that kids can put on some water shoes and wade out into the cascading pools created by the water.

Paddlers camping at the state-forest campground find themselves in the middle of the finest water for canoeing and kayaking on the Ocqueoc. The entire length of the river—beginning as far upstream as its source, Lake Emma (17 miles south)—is accessible by boat, especially in the spring, but many folks rent canoes and put in near Millersburg. Between Millersburg and Lake Huron lie 20 miles of river, with plenty of action for intermediate paddlers. Though never producing whitewater, the river does offer some fast technical turns, and at least one section needs to be portaged or waded in low water.

Anglers will find the upper portions of the Ocqueoc are warmer than the sections downstream of the falls. Dams upstream warm the river and support fishery of pike and smallmouth bass. Where cold-water streams feed the river—from the falls to Lake Huron—you will find trout and steelhead.

The campground and day-use area were built in 1976 to commemorate the country's bicentennial. The development included the Bicentennial Pathway, a long loop with two cutbacks, giving you the option of a short, medium, or long hike. The best section for viewing the falls is the shorter of the paths, which comes up just shy of crossing the Little Ocqueoc. Just downstream from the falls, the river drops into a rocky gorge with walls some 20 feet high. This trail takes you by the falls and along this stretch of river. Simply gorgeous.

Open to both hikers and mountain bikers, the longer path takes in the entire 6-mile oblong loop, hemmed in on the west by the river and on the east by Silver Creek Road. With an easy grade, the path is no push-over ride for cyclists (6 miles is 6 miles, after all), but neither will anyone with experience go home with shaky knees and sore thighs.

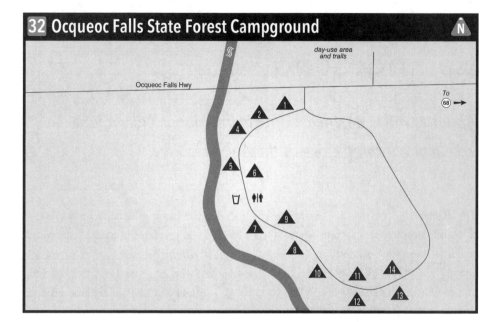

:: Getting There

From I-75, take Exit 310 for M 68 east. Follow M 68 for 30 miles, passing through Onaway on the way. The road will make a sharp 90-degree turn to the north, and then, a few miles later, turn sharply east. Ocqueoc Falls Highway is on the left just after the second turn. Turn left (west) and the campground and day-use area are less than a half mile away.

GPS COORDINATES   N45° 23.706'   W84° 03.378'

Jones Lake State Forest Campground

About 14 miles northeast of Grayling, Jones Lake offers
excellent camping close to the Au Sable River.

At the end of the day, a successful camping trip is one where all included can find something to keep themselves occupied. Maybe the camp stove ran out of fuel, the ice in the cooler melted, and you had to eat dry cereal all week. Maybe the dog got skunked. Maybe it rained and the tent leaked. All of these make for great stories to tell over future campfires. On the other hand, if campers in your party spend the week whining about being bored, you will come home only with a lesson learned—even if what you learned is who not to take camping next time.

With this in mind, Jones Lake presents a bit of a challenge. The campground sits on the southeastern shore of Jones Lake. The lake itself is a fine body of water. A total of 42.5 acres of natural lake empty directly into the East Branch of the Au Sable River. At its deepest, the lake only goes 37 feet, but having been stocked since the middle of the last century, Jones Lake is considered good fishing. Anglers regularly land largemouth bass, northern pike, and walleye, in addition to the usual bluegill and sunfish. Gas motors are not permitted on the lake, but electric trolling motors are allowed. Many folks simply cast a line from shore or wade near the perimeter.

The campground's 42 sites are organized into six loops. Loops 5 and 6 back up onto County Road 612. It's not a busy highway, but there is more traffic noise in this part of the camp than any other. The remaining loops front the lake. I think Loop 3 is the best of the lot, particularly if you can land a site on the water side of the circle. Of course, drinking water and toilets are less convenient to these sites, but they are worth the sacrifice.

The campground doesn't offer much if fishing isn't your thing. No hiking trails pass through, for example. But there is an

:: Ratings

BEAUTY: ★ ★ ★ ★
PRIVACY: ★ ★ ★
SPACIOUSNESS: ★ ★ ★ ★
QUIET: ★ ★ ★
SECURITY: ★ ★ ★ ★
CLEANLINESS: ★ ★ ★ ★ ★

:: Key Information

ADDRESS: 4216 Ranger Road, Grayling, MI 48738

OPERATED BY: Michigan DNR–Hartwick Pines State Park

CONTACT: 989-348-7068; tinyurl.com/ler867n

OPEN: Year-round, maintained May–October

SITES: 42

EACH SITE: Picnic table, fire pit

ASSIGNMENT: First come, first served

REGISTRATION: Self-register at campground.

FACILITIES: Hand-pumped water and vault toilets

PARKING: At site

FEE: $13

ELEVATION: 1,216 feet

RESTRICTIONS:

■ **Pets:** On leash only

■ **Fires:** Fire pits only

■ **Vehicles:** 2 per site; Michigan Recreation Passport required

■ **Other:** 14-day stay limit

impressive state park just a few miles away. The largest state park in the Lower Peninsula, Hartwick Pines has a full complement of outdoor recreation. It has hiking, biking, geocaching, and interpretive programs. The visitor center teaches guests about the state's lumber industry, and a logging museum commemorates that industry's history. The centerpiece of the park, however, is the Old Growth Forest Trail. It's one of the park's shortest trails—only 1.25 miles—but it takes you through 85 acres of old-growth forest. That's 85 acres of virgin white pine, the largest such stand of trees in the Lower Peninsula.

The trail is paved and accessible to wheelchairs and strollers. Beneath the towering canopy of trees, the woods are shady and generally cool. In the middle of the forest is the Chapel in the Pines. Erected in 1952, the hand-built chapel is a popular place for small weddings, though it primarily serves as a place for visitors to rest and contemplate the trees.

Those interested in a longer walk should check out the Weary Legs Trail. Hikers have opportunities along the way to make a shorter loop, but those who go all the way will walk 7.5 miles through woods and a large swath of stump fields.

The state park is responsible for maintaining the campground at Jones Lake—a welcome change from the days the forest campground was under the management of the local field office—but Hartwick Pines also has a modern campground of its own with 100 sites. The road through the campground is paved, as are the parking areas at each site. If you are okay with campers and RVs, hot showers, and flush toilets, then this just might be the place for you.

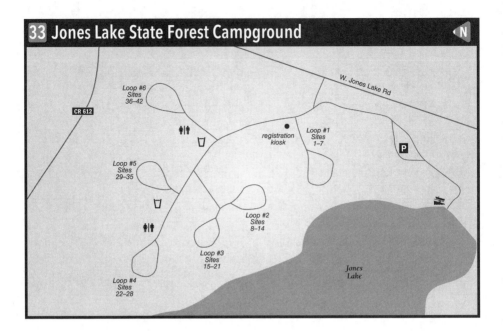

:: Getting There

From I-75, take Exit 259 north of Grayling for M 93 east. Continue 6 miles; then turn east on West County Road 612. After 3 miles, you will come to East Jones Lake Road. Turn right (south). The campground entrance is less than a quarter mile down on your right.

GPS COORDINATES   N44° 46.957'   W84° 35.263'

Upper
Peninsula

34

Brevoort Lake National Forest Campground

Brevoort Lake is known for its fishing and is considered by many to be one of the state's finest fishing lakes.

From the bridge to Naubinway, US 2 follows the gentle northwesterly curve of Lake Michigan. At first, the route's main attractions are the Weird Michigan Wax Museum, the curiously enduring Mystery Spot, and numerous places selling sandwiches, exotic jerky, and views of the straits. The bridge serves as a gateway, and businesses do a brisk trade welcoming travelers to the Upper Peninsula and offering folks on their way home a last chance at vacation memories. The commercial strip doesn't last, however, and soon passengers on westbound US 2 look out their windows to see miles of sandy Lake Michigan beach. Each summer, thousands of visitors get no farther into the Upper Peninsula than this.

:: Ratings

BEAUTY: ★ ★ ★ ★ ★
PRIVACY: ★ ★ ★ ★
SPACIOUSNESS: ★ ★ ★ ★ ★
QUIET: ★ ★ ★ ★ ★
SECURITY: ★ ★ ★ ★ ★
CLEANLINESS: ★ ★ ★ ★ ★

They find a place to hole up at night and spend their days soaking up the sun.

And there are certainly a lot of places to stay. Hotels and motels in St. Ignace are just 30 minutes away, of course, but the Hiawatha National Forest and Lake Superior State Forest maintain a mess of campgrounds, all close by. The most popular has to be the national forest's Brevoort Lake Campground. Located on a small point that separates Boedne Bay from the rest of this stunning inland lake, the unit offers 70 sites. Most are available on a first-come, first-serve basis, but the campground does set aside a small number that can be reserved. This close to Lake Michigan and the bridge, the campground stays busy throughout the summer. But, if you can't find a site here, you can always try Little Brevoort, which is the state-forest campground next door, or any one of the public campgrounds along US 2, including the Foley Creek National Forest Campground north of St. Ignace and the Straits State Park—all decent options.

The first 49 sites on Brevoort Lake thread their way up and around the spit

:: Key Information

ADDRESS: 1798 West US 2, St. Ignace, MI 49781	**REGISTRATION:** Self-register at campground.
OPERATED BY: Hiawatha National Forest, St. Ignace Ranger District	**FACILITIES:** Pressurized drinking water from a spigot and modern restrooms
CONTACT: 906-643-7900; tinyurl.com/kz9pjmp	**PARKING:** At site
OPEN: Mid-May–mid-September	**FEE:** $18
SITES: 70	**ELEVATION:** 630 feet
EACH SITE: Picnic table, fire pit with grill, and lantern post	**RESTRICTIONS:**
ASSIGNMENT: First come, first served; reservations can be made online at **recreation.gov.**	■ **Pets:** On leash only ■ **Fires:** Fire pits only ■ **Vehicles:** 2 per site

of land that inserts itself between Boedne Bay and the lake. The remaining 21 sites can be found along the south shore of the bay. Most of the sites here, 39 all tallied, are on the water, and only a dozen on the peninsula lie on the inside of the loop. The property is wooded throughout, and each site comes prepped for campers with a wooden picnic table, a fire pit with an iron grill, and a lantern post. Flush toilets and drinking water can be found in convenient locations throughout the camp.

Next to the day-use area, a camp store sells groceries and other necessities, including fishing gear. It also rents boats and canoes. Anglers will find the staff helpful. Brevoort Lake is known for its fishing and is considered by many to be one of the state's finest fishing lakes. At 4,233 acres, the lake is large and also shallow, 10–30 feet deep. Anglers can

hunt the day away—looking for the best spot—without bumping into each other. Walleye are prime targets for the casters who troll the lake (the Forest Service built a large walleye-spawning reef here years back), but folks also pull in smallmouth bass, perch, panfish, and northern pike.

The campground doesn't offer much in the way of hiking. A half-mile Ridge Interpretive Trail leads walkers up a dune and has views of Lake Michigan, but it takes all of 20 minutes to complete. Driving into the camp, you may notice a trail crossing the road that offers the promise of serious hiking. The North Country Trail (NCT) crosses east to west here before turning north toward Tahquamenon. The NCT is no day hike and comes with no convenient way to loop back home, but hikers might enjoy doing an out-and-back on a portion of this cross-country trail.

For swimming, the sandy beach that borders the eastern shore of the peninsula can be a happy alternative to the Great Lake—the waters of Lake Michigan are slow to warm in summer, but inland lakes are quicker to grab hold of and hold on to the heat. That said, the nearby stretch of Lake Michigan is beautiful, especially when enjoyed from the dunes that separate the larger lake from Brevoort Lake. In the summer, cars line up, parked alongside US 2. Yet the beach is never crowded and always has room for sunbathers to spread out.

Farther west along the highway, you come to the mouth of the Cut River. The water flows down a tall gorge. If you're not paying attention, you may not even notice that the ground has continued to rise above lake level. By the time you cross the Cut River Bridge, the idea of a river flowing 147 feet below seems a little odd. Picnic areas at both ends of the bridge allow you to get out of the car, stretch your legs, and explore this interesting structure. Then start the descent. Staircases on either side take you down to the water. Trails follow the river and lead you out to another beautiful beach on Lake Michigan.

For more wilderness and a chance at some river fishing, the South Branch of the Carp River flows west to east and through the Mackinac Wilderness, which is just a few miles north of Brevoort Lake. The wetlands bordering the river comprise much of this 12,000-acre preserve. With no roads and no footpaths, most visitors only experience the wilderness by paddling in on the Carp River or as they travel the St. Ignace–Trout Lake Rail Trail, which runs alongside M 123.

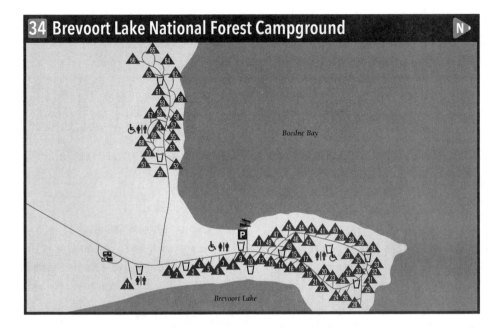

:: Getting There

From the Mackinac Bridge, follow US 2 almost exactly 17 miles to Forest Service Road 3108. There's a sign here for the campground. Turn right (north) and follow the road 1.2 miles to the campground entrance.

GPS COORDINATES   N46° 00.582'   W84° 58.278'

35

Big Knob State Forest Campground

This area is known for its dunes and swales, and lakeside sites access the beach by way of trails that lead out to the shore through low bushes and dune grass.

Big Knob Road is a narrow dirt path that wanders so much that you might be justified in questioning the sobriety of the surveyors who plotted it. As the arrow flies, the Big Knob State Forest Campground at the road's end is a little more than 4 miles south. By car it's closer to 6. After hours of wading through the beginning-of-weekend summer traffic, leaving US 2 can be a jolt to the system. And when the road hasn't been recently graded, the drive offers plenty more jolts, this time of the variety that loosen the muffler and unseat carefully packed gear. But the campers who come here seeking solitude and a quiet stretch of beach know what they're about.

:: Ratings

BEAUTY: ★ ★ ★ ★ ★
PRIVACY: ★ ★ ★ ★
SPACIOUSNESS: ★ ★ ★ ★
QUIET: ★ ★ ★ ★
SECURITY: ★ ★ ★ ★ ★
CLEANLINESS: ★ ★ ★ ★

Located on the lake-edge boundary of a large swath of Lake Superior State Forest, the rustic campground here is one of the most ignored treasures on Lake Michigan. Twenty-three sites fill out the oddly B-shaped site map. Those closest to the water, sites 1–7, sit back from the shore a bit behind a low foredune. This area is known for its dunes and swales, and lakeside sites access the beach by way of trails that lead out to the shore through low bushes and dune grass, and over a boardwalk that crosses the low wet sections.

Sites farther from the water sit in a forest made up primarily of pine. These are roomy spots with long gravel spurs that push the actual camping area back from the road. Water is available near the parking area from a hand pump, and the facilities include two outhouses—one for men, the other for women—at the far end of each loop. These are classic state-forest toilets: narrow and tall, with translucent green plastic roofs (for light). These are cleaner than most, but they still have that airline-restroom feel, and there's always

:: Key Information

ADDRESS: 5100 M 28, Newberry, MI 49868

OPERATED BY: Newberry Operations Service Center

CONTACT: 906-293-5131; tinyurl.com/27pkaur

OPEN: Year-round, though snow will prevent access in winter

SITES: 23

EACH SITE: Picnic table and fire pit

ASSIGNMENT: First come, first served

REGISTRATION: Self-register at campground.

FACILITIES: Hand-pumped potable water and vault toilets

PARKING: At site

FEE: $13

ELEVATION: 589 feet

RESTRICTIONS:

■ **Pets:** On leash only

■ **Fires:** Fire pits only

■ **Vehicles:** 2 per site; Michigan Recreation Passport required

the worry that you might stumble and accidentally tip the things over.

The day-use area is used mostly by people who have come for the trails or for a low-key place for swimming. Anglers may stay and cast their lines on a few nearby inland lakes or even use the campground as a base camp for wider excursions. From the campground, you are close to a couple of trails that explore the local geography—in particular, the Big Knob–Crow Lake Foot Trails and the Marsh Lake Foot Trail. The 1.5-mile Marsh Lake hike leads through and around the lake and its attendant bogs. The trailhead begins at the parking area in the campground, heading out to the southwest.

The trailhead for Big Knob and Crow Lake are just off Big Knob Road, north of the campground a ways. (The trail is well posted.) The shortest hike takes you 0.3

mile up to the top of Big Knob itself. This short out-and-back is worthwhile for the view. On the other side of the street, the trail dives back into the woods for a 2.5-mile loop through old dunes and marsh, passing close to Crow Lake. The trail ends at a logging road that connects back to Big Knob Road.

These hikes put the area's unique ecology on display. You might see, for example, pitcher thistles, which make their home in the dunes around the upper Great Lakes. Dwarf lake irises are another rare find. These purple flowers with deep yellow accents are only found on the northern shores of Lakes Michigan and Huron. In 1998, this iris was named the official state wildflower. Another flower, Houghton's goldenrod, grows primarily around the straits area of northern Lakes Huron and Michigan.

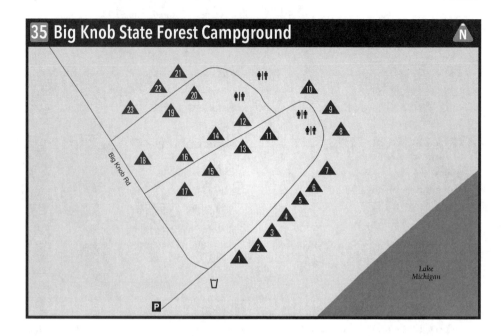

The wetlands are a favorite with birds. Visitors often see ducks and terns, in addition to the ubiquitous seagulls, near the small dune ponds. Common loons are, um, common this far north, and campers who keep an eye on the sky may see bald eagles.

A bit farther afield, a nice out-and-back hike begins east of Scott Point and takes you west to Birch Point. The author of *Hiking Michigan's Upper Peninsula,* Eric Hansen, called this "arguably some of the most remote mainland shoreline on Lake Michigan." Hikers basically walk the shoreline, which includes dunes, rocky beach, long stretches of bedrock, and immense boulders. The hike begins at the Gould City Township Park at the southernmost end of Gould City Road. Following the lake west, the trek will take you about 2.5 miles to Birch Point. Interestingly, standing on the shore here, you are closer to Beaver Island than any other spot on Michigan's mainland.

:: Getting There

From US 2 in Naubinway, drive west 7.6 miles to Big Knob Road. Take the road south about 6 miles to the campground. You can't miss it.

GPS COORDINATES   N46° 02.340'   W85° 35.634'

36

Monocle Lake National Forest Campground

From the bluff you will be able to see Canada in the distance and Whitefish Bay, as well as ships entering and leaving the St. Mary's River.

A **20-mile stretch** of West Lakeshore Drive (also known as Iroquois Road), a route beginning just west of Brimley that ends at M 123, has been designated as the Whitefish Bay Scenic Byway. It's noted particularly for various recreational opportunities and sites of historical importance: a typical itinerary might include stopping at Brimley State Park, fishing or kayaking in Whitefish Bay, visiting the Bay Mills Reservation, touring the Point Iroquois Lighthouse, and camping next to Monocle Lake.

Between Bay Mills and Point Iroquois on Lake Superior's Whitefish Bay,

you will find two small inland lakes. The southernmost of the pair is a smallish body of water nearly bisected by a thin point, the aptly named Spectacle Lake. A short ways to the northwest is its neighbor, the oblong Monocle Lake. Behind the lakes, running parallel with the shore of the bay, a tall ridge rises from the forest, creating a scenic backdrop.

The campground on Monocle Lake is part of the Hiawatha National Forest. Most of the sites are nestled in a sprawling stand of tall maples. Other trees include aspens and white birches. The road through the camp is paved, and most sites are floored in packed dirt. None of the sites front the lake, though a few—sites 29 and 30, for example—sit directly across the road from the water and offer nice views. I also liked sites 13–16. These are found on the forest side of the campground, surrounded by maples, with plenty of privacy. Facilities include drinking water and vault toilets but no showers.

:: Ratings

BEAUTY: ★ ★ ★ ★ ★
PRIVACY: ★ ★ ★ ★
SPACIOUSNESS: ★ ★ ★ ★
QUIET: ★ ★ ★ ★ ★
SECURITY: ★ ★ ★ ★ ★
CLEANLINESS: ★ ★ ★ ★ ★

:: Key Information

ADDRESS: 4000 I-75 Business Spur, Sault Ste. Marie, MI 49783

OPERATED BY: Hiawatha National Forest, Sault Ste. Marie Ranger District

CONTACT: 906-635-5311; tinyurl.com/qeo39wu

OPEN: Mid-May–mid-October

SITES: 39

EACH SITE: Picnic table, fire pit, and lantern post

ASSIGNMENT: First come, first served

REGISTRATION: Self-register at campground.

FACILITIES: Pressurized water and vault toilets

PARKING: At site

FEE: $16

ELEVATION: 652 feet

RESTRICTIONS:
- **Pets:** On leash only
- **Fires:** Fire pits only
- **Vehicles:** 2 per site

The day-use part of the facility includes a picnic area, a boat launch, a swimming beach, and a decent little nature hike. The lake is the big attraction. At 172 acres, this respectable lake counters its size with surprising depth (up to 55 feet) and great scenery. Private property makes up its north end, but all along its western shore is that impressive ridge I mentioned before. Its south end features a sandy beach, offering a somewhat warmer alternative to a dip in Lake Superior. Anglers casting a line here—from a boat or the park's fishing pier—pull in northern pike, smallmouth bass, and yellow perch. The Michigan Department of Natural Resources watches the walleye population closely and stocks the lake with the fish in hopes of creating a sustainable population.

The Monocle Lake Loop Trail leads hikers through 2 miles of a northern hardwood forest. The trail begins as a level path, accessible to visitors using wheelchairs. As the trail crosses wetlands, a boardwalk keeps your feet dry. A beaver dam along the way would be of special interest to kids, and you might also see blue herons by the water and ospreys diving toward the lake for fish. After about a quarter mile, the trail leads up to a scenic overlook. This is where the sweet innocence of this stroll through the woods takes a serious turn. It's a steep, strenuous climb to the top, but, from the bluff, you will be able to see Canada in the distance and Whitefish Bay, as well as ships entering and leaving the St. Mary's River. This stunning view makes the climb worthwhile.

Beyond the campground, be sure to take in some of the historical sites. Just up the road, the Point Iroquois Lighthouse guides ships entering the St. Mary's River. The point is named for an event that took place here in the late 1600s. The Iroquois people hold a significant place in the history of upstate New York and in the colonial wars in America and Canada. Though their influence extends farther east in Canada and on Lake Ontario, the Iroquois name is not bandied about much in Michigan. Back in 1662, as the Iroquois were looking to expand their territory into the Great Lakes, they sent a war party west to the shores of Whitefish Bay. The Ojibwa living in this region discovered that the group was camped on this point and attacked. The Iroquois were wiped out after a day of fighting, and this battle became the last in a series that ended the Iroquois's ambitions for this territory.

About 200 years later, a lighthouse was erected on the point. When you visit today, you see the lighthouse and residence that were built in 1870 to replace the original tower. A visit to the lighthouse should include taking some time to stroll through the maritime museum there, which is maintained by the Bay Mills–Brimley Historical Research Society.

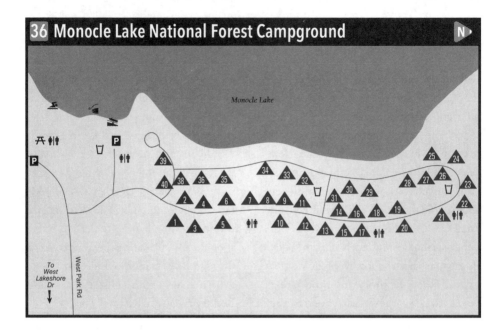

:: Getting There

From I-75, get off at Exit 386 for M 28 heading west. After 7.5 miles, turn north on M 221 toward Brimley. Once through town, turn left at the T. You're now on West Lakeshore Drive/Iroquois Road. At 6.2 miles, you will see the sign for the campground. Turn left onto West Park Road, and follow that into the camp.

GPS COORDINATES   N46° 28.224'   W84° 38.358'

37

Bay View National Forest Campground

The sandy beach attracts more sunbathers and rock hunters than it does swimmers; though, if you can take the temperature, this is a great place for a swim.

Consider this: every year an average of 10,000 ships pass through the locks in Sault Ste. Marie, and that's only April–December, when the passage isn't closed due to ice. (A dramatic rise in the temperature of Lake Superior in recent years may mean that the locks will stay open longer in the future.) This number includes everything from Soo Locks tour boats to pleasure craft to the Great Lakes freighters (the workhorses of freshwater shipping). The freighters are the largest ships on the freshwater seas, and the largest of these are the thousand-footers that can carry more than 88,000 tons of cargo.

There are many great reasons to come to the Upper Peninsula—hunting

and fishing, snowmobiling and dogsledding, fancy casinos, and some nice golf courses—but there is a certain pleasure in simply setting up a chair overlooking Lake Superior and watching the ships go by. From your campsite at Bay View Campground on the southern shore of Whitefish Bay, you can watch the biggest of these, the freighters (those sweetwater titans), make way for either the downlake passage toward Lake Huron or out into the open waters of Lake Superior.

Located on West Lakeshore Drive (or Iroquois Road, depending on your map), the campground is part of the Whitefish Bay Scenic Byway. Sites worth visiting along the way include Point Iroquois Lighthouse to the east, the nearby Big Pine Day Use Area, and the Monocle Lake Campground and Recreation Area (covered on page 147).

Bay View has 25 sites. The layout is simple enough—the campground is essentially a long one-way pulloff from the main road. All but nine of the sites overlook Lake Superior from a low,

:: Ratings

BEAUTY: ★ ★ ★ ★ ★
PRIVACY: ★ ★ ★ ★
SPACIOUSNESS: ★ ★ ★ ★ ★
QUIET: ★ ★ ★ ★
SECURITY: ★ ★ ★ ★
CLEANLINESS: ★ ★ ★ ★ ★

:: Key Information

ADDRESS: 4000 I-75 Business Spur, Sault Ste. Marie, MI 49783

OPERATED BY: Hiawatha National Forest, Sault Ste. Marie Ranger District

CONTACT: 906-635-5311; **tinyurl.com/oruc436**

OPEN: Mid-May–mid-October

SITES: 25

EACH SITE: Picnic table, fire pit with grill, and lantern post

ASSIGNMENT: First come, first served; reservations can be made online at **recreation.gov.**

REGISTRATION: Self-register at campground.

FACILITIES: Drinking water and vault toilets

PARKING: At site

FEE: $16

ELEVATION: 614 feet

RESTRICTIONS:

■ **Pets:** On leash only

■ **Fires:** Fire pits only

■ **Vehicles:** 2 per site

wooded bluff. Down below, a sandy beach attracts more sunbathers and rock hunters than it does swimmers; though, if you can take the temperature, this is a great place for a swim. Vault toilets (some quite new) and access to water from hand pumps are staggered throughout the length of the camp. There's hardly a place here where you'd find the facilities inconvenient, whether during the day or stumbling through the dark late at night.

The sites here can accommodate trailers and small RVs. Heavily wooded with tall, thick pines and a mix of northern hardwoods, the hill down to the water is covered in lichens and ferns. Take a quick look at the campground's list of sites and the official count, and you will notice that one seems to be missing. Site 7 was recently removed to make room for a new vault toilet. This wasn't one of the lakefront sites, and the newer additions of sites

25 and 26 more than make up for its loss.

In fact, these two new sites are perhaps the best of the bunch. At the west end of the campground, a small parking area, just enough for several cars, marks the entrance to sites 25 and 26. These spacious walk-in sites put tent campers as far from the vagaries of less courteous neighbors as is possible in a campground setting. Like the rest, these sites are set up with a picnic table, fire pit, and lantern post. The lots are grassy, and a thinning of the trees allows for better views of the water.

In the summer, camp hosts occupy one of the sites. These folks are always good to have around and good to know. Often, hosts will return to the same campground year after year, giving the place some consistency. They carry with them the memories of past summers and are your best resource when it comes time to explore the area.

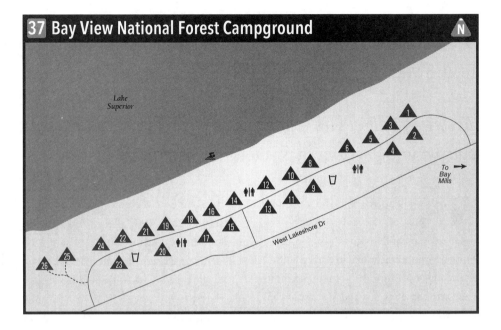

37 Bay View National Forest Campground

Along Lakeshore Drive, the road passes over numerous rivers and streams, all draining into the bay. Anglers catch lake trout and salmon near the bridges that span the flowing water. They also do well at nearby Monocle Lake. Ask the host about the best places to put in a boat or park for access to these flowing waters.

One mile east of Bay View, the Hiawatha National Forest maintains an excellent picnic area. The Big Pine Day Use Area sits on a low sandy bluff, overlooking Lake Superior and a beautiful stretch of beach. The spot's most distinguishing feature is the stand of tall pines towering above, under which you will find a number of picnic tables liberally distributed. Check with the U.S. Forest Service about other public beaches along this part of the bay.

:: Getting There

From I-75, get off at Exit 386 for M 28 heading west. After 7.5 miles, turn north on M 221 toward Brimley. Once through town, turn left at the T. You're now on West Lakeshore Drive/Iroquois Road. After driving about 15 miles, you will see the sign for the campground. Turn right into the camp.

GPS COORDINATES N46° 26.976' W84° 46.872'

38

Tahquamenon Falls State Park:
RIVERMOUTH PINES CAMPGROUND

The Rivermouth Pines Campground offers the most secluded and picturesque campsites you will find in the park.

Nothing about the upper or lower sections of the Tahquamenon—a quiet river, meandering yet ponderous—hints at the cataclysms in the middle. Springing up from the Tahquamenon Lakes, the river is steeped in tannins as it flows through cedar bogs, giving it a unique copper tone (locals sometimes call it Root Beer Falls). The more dramatic of the two sections, the Upper Falls sends water over a 48-foot drop. At this point the river has expanded to more than 200 feet, creating a wide curtain of falling water. The Lower Falls farther downstream are a combination of five smaller cascades, which are a bit more approachable.

The state park here has three campgrounds—Upper Falls, Lower Falls, and,

:: Ratings

BEAUTY: ★ ★ ★ ★ ★
PRIVACY: ★ ★ ★
SPACIOUSNESS: ★ ★ ★ ★ ★
QUIET: ★ ★ ★
SECURITY: ★ ★ ★ ★ ★
CLEANLINESS: ★ ★ ★ ★ ★

several miles to the east, the Rivermouth Campground. The falls are one of the state's biggest attractions, up there with Mackinac Island, Sleeping Bear Dunes, and Pictured Rocks. Even downstaters who cross the bridge on rare occasions will make a pilgrimage to Tahquamenon at some point, if even just for the kids. All of these visitors stop by the Upper Falls parking lot for the short hike to the observation platform. Many stay on to spend money on park concessions, and some even come to camp.

Rivermouth has both a modern section (Rivermouth Modern) and a semimodern section (Rivermouth Pines). Choose the latter. Off by itself, the Rivermouth Pines Campground offers the most secluded and picturesque campsites you will find in the park. The road through the semimodern campground parallels the gentle curve of the Tahquamenon River. For most of its length, the campground has sites on both sides of the road. All are great. Even campers back against the woods have a view of the water. To prevent erosion of

:: Key Information

ADDRESS: 41382 West M 123, Paradise, MI 49768

OPERATED BY: Michigan DNR–Tahquamenon Falls State Park

CONTACT: 906-492-3415; **michigan.gov/tahquamenonfalls**

OPEN: May–December (modern facilities close mid-October)

SITES: 36

EACH SITE: Picnic table and fire pit

ASSIGNMENT: Reservations can be made online at **midnrreservations.com** and by calling 800-447-2757.

REGISTRATION: Register at campground office.

FACILITIES: Water and vault toilets; flush toilets and showers available at neighboring campground

PARKING: At site

FEE: $16 ($12 off-season when modern facilities are closed)

ELEVATION: 626 feet

RESTRICTIONS:

■ **Pets:** On leash only

■ **Fires:** Fire pits only

■ **Vehicles:** Michigan Recreation Passport required

the riverbank, the park restricts access to the water to certain areas. Campers with sites on the water will have to carry canoes (and themselves) to one of these points of entry.

Sites 106 and 107 share a small clearing, surrounded by cedars and birches. A clump of trees serves as a boundary between the two sites; otherwise, they enjoy privacy from the rest of the campsites. The sites are on the wooded side of the road but have an unobstructed view of the river. Farther on (sites 120 and above), the woods open up. Plenty of trees shelter the sites, but there's less undergrowth. Amenities in the semi-modern campground include vault toilets and water from a hand-pumped well. A short walk through the woods, however, takes you to the modern campground at Rivermouth with its flush toilets and showers.

As it gets closer to Lake Superior, the river bends and winds as if trying to delay the inevitable emptying into the Great Lake. The river mouth itself is across from the campground. A small picnic area, boat launch, and fishing dock give access to the river where it meets Whitefish Bay. This small roadside park seems to be used mostly by fishermen and others looking to put a boat in the water. It's worth a visit, even a short one, to see the contrast between the steel blue of the lake as it is filled with the river's rusty water.

The North Country Trail passes through the Tahquamenon Falls State Park, linking the Rivermouth Campground with the Upper and Lower

Falls before continuing north toward Lake Superior and the Pictured Rocks National Lakeshore. But this is hardly the only opportunity to experience the wilderness areas of the state park. With more than 46,000 acres of rivers, lakes, and streams, the park has enough trails here for multiday trips into the park, and numerous loops make excellent day hikes. Even exploring the falls can turn into an opportunity for a relaxing walk in the woods—consider the 4-mile River Trail, which connects the Upper and Lower Falls.

The area's other big attraction is the wildlife. Nearby, Newberry touts itself as Michigan's Official Moose Capital, and it's not uncommon for visitors to see deer, black bears, and eagles in the park. The state publishes a moose-viewing guide, titled *Michigan Moose*, which you can pick up at the visitor center. It gives good advice on finding these animals.

Because Tahquamenon Falls State Park enjoys a steady flow of visitors throughout the summer, concessions here are particularly good. In addition to the usual snack station, you'll find the Tahquamenon Falls Brewery & Pub, a full-service sit-down restaurant, near the Upper Falls. With a surprisingly deep menu and excellent microbrews, it's one of the nicest places to eat in the area.

From the town of Paradise on M 123, it's only 10 miles to Whitefish Point. For a side trip, consider spending the day on the point exploring the Whitefish Point Lighthouse and Great Lakes Shipwreck Museum. This complex used to be a Coast Guard station, the light guiding ships around the point and into Whitefish Bay. Many know it today as the eastern end of Lake Superior's "shipwreck coast." The museum does more than just tell the stories of the ships and sailors who fell upon hard times on these lakes; it uses sound and creative lighting to take visitors down through the darkling water, giving the displays of recovered artifacts and models of shipwrecks a haunting context. Most visitors recognize the memorial to the *Edmund Fitzgerald*. In 1975, a mere 17 miles from Whitefish Bay, the freighter sank, taking with it the ship's entire crew. The museum displays the ship's 200-pound bronze bell.

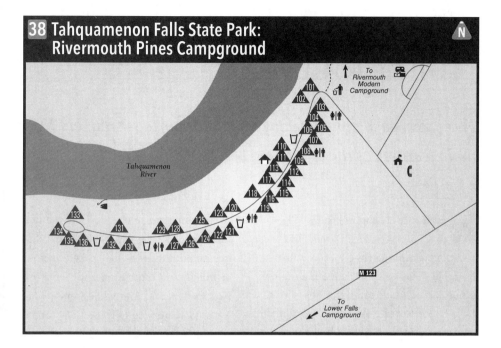

38 Tahquamenon Falls State Park: Rivermouth Pines Campground

:: Getting There

From the Mackinac Bridge, take I-75 to Exit 352. Follow M 123 north and west 50.3 miles. The campground is on your left before you cross over the Tahquamenon River (about 5 miles south of the village of Paradise).

GPS COORDINATES   N46° 33.366'   W85° 02.124'

39

Pretty Lake State Forest Campground

Five lakes, each connected by stream or portage trail, are the main features of the quiet area.

North of Newberry, from Whitefish Point across to Grand Marais and the beginning of the Pictured Rocks National Lakeshore, the state maintains a number of small campgrounds within Lake Superior State Forest. Recreational planners here have always had the wisdom to develop campgrounds near lakes and rivers. From Culhane Lake and Bodi Lake northwest of Tahquamenon to the fabled Two-Hearted River and a series of small forest lakes that stretch west almost to Munising, dozens of places to camp can be found.

While all of these campgrounds offer remote locations on scenic lakes and rivers, some are not as well maintained as others. With great trepidation I visited an outhouse on Bodi Lake, the floor of which sank more than 2 inches when I stepped inside. And while I enjoy having a good story to tell, the unfortunate chain of events I was imagining seemed like the kind of story I would rather hear from somebody else. One campground I can recommend without hesitation, however, is the Pretty Lake State Forest Campground, which is part of the greater Pretty Lake Quiet Area.

Five lakes, each connected by stream or portage trail, are the main features of the quiet area. Pretty Lake acts as a portal into this unique preserve. It is the only lake that can be accessed by car. And from here, because motorized boats are prohibited on all the lakes, the only way to explore the area is under your own power. The main campground lies on the northern edge of the lake.

The campground has 18 sites arranged around three loops, about half a dozen of which sit on the water. Facing

:: Ratings

> BEAUTY: ★ ★ ★ ★
> PRIVACY: ★ ★ ★ ★ ★
> SPACIOUSNESS: ★ ★ ★ ★
> QUIET: ★ ★ ★ ★ ★
> SECURITY: ★ ★ ★ ★ ★
> CLEANLINESS: ★ ★ ★ ★

:: Key Information

ADDRESS: 30042 CR 407, Newberry, MI 49868

OPERATED BY: Michigan DNR–Muskallonge Lake State Park

CONTACT: 906-658-3338; tinyurl.com/2g9aagq

OPEN: Year-round, though snow will prevent access in winter

SITES: 23

EACH SITE: Picnic table and fire pit

ASSIGNMENT: First come, first served

REGISTRATION: Self-register at campground.

FACILITIES: Hand-pumped potable water and vault toilets

PARKING: At site (parking lot for walk-in sites)

FEE: $13

ELEVATION: 760 feet

RESTRICTIONS:

■ **Pets:** On leash only

■ **Fires:** Fire pits only

■ **Vehicles:** 2 per site; Michigan Recreation Passport required

south toward the lake, these sites allow you to take full advantage of the sun, which can sit pretty low, even in the early and late summer, in these latitudes. Each site is equipped with a wooden picnic table and a fire pit. The vault toilets are on the old side but well maintained.

Beyond these 18, the campground has an additional 5 walk-in sites that offer campers a mini backpacking or wilderness-canoeing adventure. Purely rustic by design, these remote campsites can be found west of Pretty Lake on Camp Eight Lake and Beaverhouse Lake. A trail less than a mile long leads hikers from the parking area near the Pretty Lake boat launch to the sites. Or paddlers can load up their gear in a canoe and get to the sites by water. In keeping with a true canoe-camping experience,

the area's lakes are connected with portages (the longest: a 250-foot hike between Camp Eight and Beaverhouse).

Anglers can spend days exploring these lakes. Deep, crystal-clear waters are bordered by a forest of white pines and mixed hardwoods. Deadfall trees along the shore create the perfect habitat for bass. Pretty Lake is on the smallish side. Its 47 acres go deep, however—well over 60 feet deep on the western half of the lake. An able angler should find splake, walleye, and yellow perch. (If you haven't heard of splake, it is the offspring of a male brook trout, also called a speckled trout, and a female lake trout.)

At its deepest, Camp Eight Lake is more than 70 feet. Folks catch rainbow trout, yellow perch, and smallmouth bass. Beaverhouse Lake, also more than

60 feet deep, is known for largemouth bass, walleye, sunfish, and yellow perch.

If your interest leans more toward fly-fishing, you might want to ditch the lakes altogether. Camping at Pretty Lake puts you in easy reach of one of the Upper Peninsula's more famous rivers. Of Ernest Hemingway's short stories, best known perhaps are those that feature his protagonist Nick Adams, who is often a thinly veiled characterization of the author himself. The two-part story that finishes the collection *In Our Time* is titled "Big Two-Hearted River." Hemingway knew the rivers of northern Michigan and found a bit of poetry in the name. In all likelihood, the actual river described in the story is the Fox River, 20 miles or so to the west, but the poetry of the Two-Hearted continues to captivate.

Close to Pretty Lake, three state-forest campgrounds—High Bridge, Reed and Green Bridge, and Mouth of the Two-Hearted River—sit alongside this fabled water. Six miles northeast of High Bridge, paddlers can still find the Two-Hearted River Canoe Campground. Though no longer maintained, it is still within the state forest, where wilderness-camping rules apply. In addition to the campgrounds on the river, the state forest maintains another half dozen within a short drive. All would be okay alternatives to Pretty Lake, if you want to stay close to the river for early-morning casts.

Hikers looking to stretch their legs will find that the North Country Trail passes just 5 miles north of the Pretty Lake State Forest Campground. If more noise and speed are what you need, the Pine Ridge Trail and the Two-Hearted Trail for off-road vehicles lie to the north and northeast, respectively. For families looking for more beach, Muskallonge State Park, 8 miles north, straddles the shore of Lake Superior and Muskallonge Lake. While the Great Lake is often too cold for swimming, Muskallonge has a decent swimming beach on warmer water.

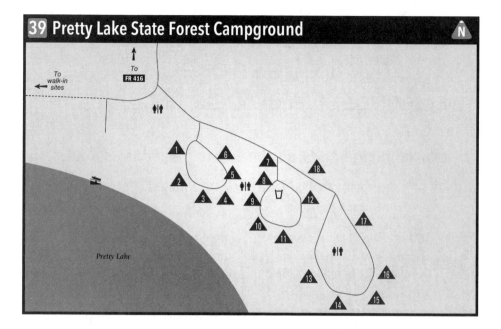

39 Pretty Lake State Forest Campground

To walk-in sites

To FR 416

Pretty Lake

:: Getting There

Just over 4.5 miles north of the center of Newberry at Fourmile Corner, turn left (west) on CR 407 (also called H 37). Follow the road 17.5 miles (after the first 4 miles, it turns north). Turn left (west again) on FR 416. On maps, the road is also called Holland Lake Road and Stellwagon Road. Keep heading west 2.7 miles. The long drive to the campground is on the south side of the road.

GPS COORDINATES   N46° 36.237'   W85° 39.483'

40

Pictured Rocks National Lakeshore:

TWELVEMILE BEACH CAMPGROUND

If you're going to hoof it all the way to the Pictured Rocks, a view of Lake Superior should not be missed.

The **Upper** Peninsula is bounded to the north by the lake the French called le lac supérieur. The Ojibwa simply called it kitchi-gami, or "the great lake." And with his attempt at translating Finnish folk poetry into the American experience, Henry Wadsworth Longfellow called it Big-Sea-Water in *The Song of Hiawatha*. Lake Superior, it seems, needs no fancy label. It is enough to behold the lake and simply say, "Wow, that's a big body of water." And it is. It is the largest of the Great Lakes in terms of both acreage and depth.

It wasn't until the 1730s that a sailing ship was seen on Lake Superior. Native peoples traveled by canoe and taught the Europeans to do the same. Often, they paddled the two-person birchbark canoes you imagine, but the voyageurs transported furs in boats 35 feet long. Traveling along the southern shore of Lake Superior presented a particular challenge—a 12-mile stretch of cliffs that offered no safe harbor. It could take several hours to traverse the length of what we now call the Pictured Rocks, plenty of time for an unfortunate change in the weather. As such, the sight of these inspiring sandstone cliffs, with their undulating bands of color, struck in early travelers a sense of urgency if not fear.

Pictured Rocks National Lakeshore encompasses 42 miles of the Lake Superior shoreline, including these famed cliffs. Inland, it includes 11,740 acres of woods, waterfalls, and lakes. This national park has three campgrounds—Hurricane River, Twelvemile Beach, and Beaver Lake. Hurricane River has 21 sites on two loops. Close to Lake Superior, it is

:: Ratings

BEAUTY: ★ ★ ★ ★ ★
PRIVACY: ★ ★ ★ ★ ★
SPACIOUSNESS: ★ ★ ★ ★ ★
QUIET: ★ ★ ★ ★ ★
SECURITY: ★ ★ ★ ★ ★
CLEANLINESS: ★ ★ ★ ★ ★

:: Key Information

ADDRESS: N8391 Sand Point Road, Munising, MI 49862

OPERATED BY: Pictured Rocks National Lakeshore

CONTACT: 906-387-2607; **nps.gov/piro**

OPEN: Year-round, though not maintained in winter

SITES: 36

EACH SITE: Picnic table, fire pit, and tent pad

ASSIGNMENT: First come, first served

REGISTRATION: Self-register at campground.

FACILITIES: Drinkable water and vault toilets

PARKING: At site

FEE: $14 for camping; $16 for sites on Lake Superior

ELEVATION: 639 feet

RESTRICTIONS:

■ **Pets:** On leash only

■ **Fires:** Fire pits only

also close to Grand Marais (just 12 miles) and has trail access to the Au Sable Light Station. As such, it sees a fair amount of traffic. Near the middle of the park, eight secluded sites on a small inland lake comprise the Beaver Lake Campground. But if you're going to hoof it all the way to the Pictured Rocks, a view of Lake Superior should not be missed, which is why I suggest the 36 sites of the Twelvemile Beach Campground.

The road into the campground passes through a sprawling white-birch forest, carpeted everywhere with ferns. Once the road reaches the lake, it forks to the left and right. To the right, a small parking area gives visitors a chance to stretch their legs and perhaps walk down to the beach or hike a little of the North Country Trail. To the left, campsites are situated down the length of the dirt drive,

which has a small oblong loop at the end. High on a bluff, more than half the sites overlook Lake Superior and the beach for which the campground is named. Birches and the occasional pine provide shade.

Amenities at the park's campgrounds are limited to vault toilets and drinkable water. During the camping season, sites cost $14 per night, but $16 if you take a lakeside site at Twelvemile Beach. The campground remains open year-round, but during the colder months rangers collect no fees and the campground facilities are unavailable. In the winter, roads are often closed because of snow.

Below the campground, along the lake, Twelvemile Beach stretches from the Pictured Rocks in the west to the Grand Sable Banks near Grand Marais in the east. This beach is just one of several features worth exploring in the park—the

Grand Sable Banks and Dunes, Chapel Rock and Beach, Miners Beach and Miners River, and, for a different perspective on the Pictured Rocks themselves, Miners Castle. There are also several waterfalls to discover. Stop by one of the park's visitor centers for a map and information on trails.

Ironically, staying in the park isn't the best way to see the cliffs themselves. To really get an idea of what all the fuss is about, the Pictured Rocks should be seen from the water. One option is to bring or rent sea kayaks and paddle out on your own. This is only recommended for skilled paddlers. The water of Lake Superior can reach into the high 60s in the warmest years, but these are the extreme temperatures—the mid-50s are average for summer. And as I mentioned before, the cliffs offer no sanctuary if the water should turn rough. The easiest way to get a peek is to take one of the three-hour boat tours out of Munising offered by Pictured Rocks Cruises (906-387-3386; **picturedrocks.com**). Many travelers will begin and end their experience of the park with one of these afternoon trips. Tours leave fairly regularly in the summer from the City Dock, and the narration includes information on various formations and some history of the Pictured Rocks and nearby Grand Island.

While you're on the Munising side of the park, visit the Munising Falls Interpretive Center. From here, an 800-foot path leads to Munising Falls. Continuing deeper into the park along East Munising Avenue, turn onto Pictured Rock Trails (also called Miners Castle Road and H 11), and follow the signs to the Miners Falls. From the trailhead to the waterfall is just a 0.5-mile hike. Then keep heading north to Miners Castle, which has a picnic area and an overlook of Lake Superior and a section of the Pictured Rocks.

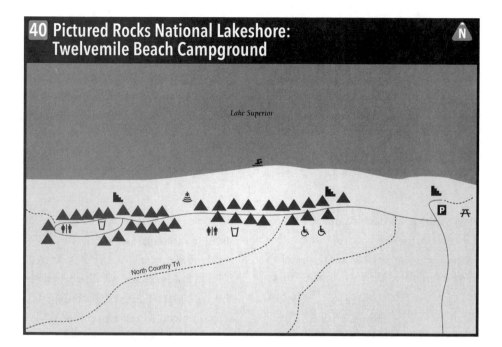

40 Pictured Rocks National Lakeshore:
Twelvemile Beach Campground

Lake Superior

North Country Trl

:: Getting There

The campgrounds at Pictured Rocks National Lakeshore are approached from the Grand Marais side of the park. From the bridge, take I-75 to Exit 352. Follow M 123 north to M 28 (about 22 miles). Turn left and continue west 46 miles. At the junction with M 77, turn right. Grand Marais is 24 miles north. Turn left on Carlson Street downtown and follow the signs to the Grand Sable Visitor Center. They can offer directions and help you get your bearings.

GPS COORDINATES   N46° 38.646'   W86° 12.318'

41

Petes Lake National Forest Campground

This campground is embraced by a forest of dark green throughout the summer.

The **Hiawatha** National Forest divides nicely into two units. The eastern portion of the forest stretches from Whitefish Bay down to the Straits of Mackinac. The western portion begins at the western edge of Pictured Rocks National Lakeshore, reaching halfway between Munising and Marquette. Its southern edge is along Lake Michigan, including the shores of Big and Little Bays de Noc and the peninsula between them. Combined, both halves total nearly 900,000 acres of forest.

Petes Lake Campground falls roughly in the center of the western unit. This part of the forest is known for dozens of small inland lakes and the Sturgeon and Indian Rivers. The area is a sportsman's

paradise, and Petes Lake offers some of its best camping. Located just 13 miles south of Munising and 25 miles north of US 2 (a few miles west of where it passes through Manistique), the campground is convenient to the Upper Peninsula's major travel routes. Yet the main road through here, H 13, is hardly a busy thoroughfare. Most traffic north and south follows M 94, and this contributes to the campground's remote feel.

Forty-seven campsites, laid out in a shape that resembles a split hot-dog bun, sit on the northern shore of Petes Lake, less than a mile east of H13. The road through the camp is paved, and the individual sites have gravel spurs.

The surrounding woods lend sites plenty of privacy. This campground is embraced by a forest of dark green throughout the summer. The two walk-in sites, 7a and 8a, make Petes Lake especially attractive. You will find parking for these sites next to the trailhead on the eastern edge of camp. The first is a short ways through the woods. Site 7a is a spacious lawn overlooking Petes Lake.

:: Ratings

BEAUTY: ★ ★ ★ ★ ★
PRIVACY: ★ ★ ★ ★ ★
SPACIOUSNESS: ★ ★ ★ ★ ★
QUIET: ★ ★ ★ ★ ★
SECURITY: ★ ★ ★ ★ ★
CLEANLINESS: ★ ★ ★ ★ ★

:: Key Information

ADDRESS: 400 East Munising Avenue, Munising, MI 49862

OPERATED BY: Hiawatha National Forest, Munising Ranger District

CONTACT: 906-387-2512; tinyurl.com/ojd6fbz

OPEN: Mid-May–late September

SITES: 47

EACH SITE: Picnic table, fire pit with grill, and lantern post

ASSIGNMENT: First come, first served; some sites can be reserved online at recreation.gov.

REGISTRATION: Self-register at campground.

FACILITIES: Drinking water and vault toilets

PARKING: At site

FEE: $16–$21

ELEVATION: 809 feet

RESTRICTIONS:

■ **Pets:** On leash only

■ **Fires:** Fire pits only

■ **Vehicles:** 2 per site

Offering little in the way of shade, the lot makes up for it with enough room for a private game of Ultimate Frisbee. The second site is found a quarter mile east and also offers a view of the lake. A stand of tall pines gives the spot the feel of a rustic hideaway.

The trail out to the sites serves another purpose as well. It is mainly used by hikers and bikers as part of the Bruno's Run Trail, a 9-mile path that connects Petes Lake with a string of neighboring lakes. Bruno's Run attracts hikers and snowshoers but is also the only single-track mountain-biking trail in the county. Backpackers making a multiday trip can stay at Petes Lake or Widewaters Campgrounds, or set up on Ewing Point. The latter spot is one of the national forest's dispersed campgrounds. The one walk-in site there features a pit toilet but no drinking water. Another option, and one that would allow you to carry less gear, would be to rent the cabin on McKeever Lake.

East of H 13, the trail winds around several lakes: Petes, McKeever, Wedge, and Dipper. Crossing to the west of H 13, the path follows the Indian River to Widewaters Campground. Leaving the river and heading north to Moccasin Lake, the trail leads through the Hemlock Cathedral—a stand of hemlocks more than a century old. From Moccasin Lake, the trail turns east back to Petes Lake. Along the way hikers walk over rolling terrain, through marsh, and across many a stream.

Mountain bikers will find the route an easy afternoon's ride. Not as technical as some of the trails you might find up near Marquette, the path still offers more challenges than people used to riding local dirt roads will be accustomed to. There are some great places to stop and rest and take in the view along the way.

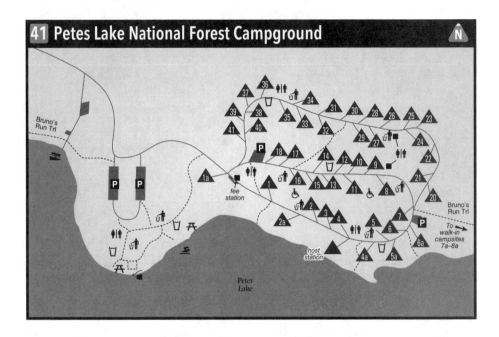

Anglers, of course, will know all about the local lakes. There are quite a few, and boat access is easy to come by. In addition to the still waters, there is also the Indian River. Paddlers and anglers alike will find Petes Lake a convenient point for accessing the river. The Widewaters Campground on Fish Lake is a fine put-in. Downstream from there you can float 36 miles of river to Indian Lake, which is northwest of Manistique—that's well over 20 hours of canoeing. (Side note: Also feeding the Indian River is Kitch-iti-kipi, meaning "big spring." At Palms Book State Park, you can take the observation raft out over the spring and look down through 40 feet of crystal-clear water.) With primitive campgrounds conveniently spaced along the route, the river would perhaps be better suited for a wilderness paddling trip.

:: Getting There

Leave I-75 at Exit 352, heading west and then north on M 123. When you come to M 28, after driving a little more than 33 miles, turn left, heading west toward Newberry. Drive 78.5 miles. Just as you enter Wetmore, turn south on H 13. At about 10 miles you will see the sign for Petes Lake–the road is on the left: Forest Service Road 2173. If you come to the sign for the Widewaters Campground, you've gone too far south.

GPS COORDINATES   N46° 13.752'   W86° 35.958'

42

Portage Bay State Forest Campground

The sandy lots are tucked behind a long, narrow foredune overgrown with cedar trees, juniper bushes, and ferns.

In all likelihood, Portage Bay got its name from early travelers who used the bay as the beginning of a shortcut across the narrowest point on the Garden Peninsula. Hiking about a mile inland from the water, groups making their way by canoe could pick up Garden Creek, which would lead them out to Garden Bay. The minor inconvenience of this short portage could save them 30 miles of open-water paddling. Many of the bays and harbors on the Great Lakes, especially those along the Upper Peninsula, bear names given them by the French. To the east is Seul Choix Point (pronounced here "sis-shwah"), which once provided a safe place for French trappers caught in a storm. They wryly called it *seul choix,* or "only choice."

:: Ratings

BEAUTY: ★ ★ ★ ★
PRIVACY: ★ ★ ★ ★ ★
SPACIOUSNESS: ★ ★ ★ ★ ★
QUIET: ★ ★ ★ ★ ★
SECURITY: ★ ★ ★ ★ ★
CLEANLINESS: ★ ★ ★ ★

I find it fascinating to walk the beach at Portage Bay State Forest Campground and contemplate what kind of men they were who found it easier to lug a canoe (which might carry a dozen men) and hundreds of pounds of furs across the Garden Peninsula than to paddle around it. The campground gives no hint of such arduous choices. At the end of a winding, narrow dirt road, far from US 2 and the civilization it offers, Portage Bay seems a world away, from both its past and our present.

Portage Bay offers 23 sites along a remote stretch of northern Lake Michigan. The sandy lots are tucked away behind a long, narrow foredune that is grown over with cedar trees, juniper bushes, ferns, and the occasional birch. The dune is not so tall; at some sites you can catch the glimmer of sunlight off the water through the trees. Other sites, such as 14, seem to wedge themselves into the sand, creating a sort of natural shelter—perfect for creating a campsite at one with the surrounding terrain.

Surrounded by a cedar forest, the sites are shady, large enough to spread

:: Key Information

ADDRESS: 4785 II Road, Garden, MI 49835	**FACILITIES:** Hand-pumped potable water and pit toilets
OPERATED BY: Michigan DNR–Fayette Historic State Park	**PARKING:** At site
CONTACT: 906-644-2603; tinyurl.com/2uh85qy	**FEE:** $13
OPEN: Year-round, though snow will prevent access in winter	**ELEVATION:** 586 feet
SITES: 23	**RESTRICTIONS:**
EACH SITE: Picnic table and fire pit	■ **Pets:** On leash only
ASSIGNMENT: First come, first served	■ **Fires:** Fire pits only
REGISTRATION: Self-register on-site	■ **Vehicles:** 2 per site; Michigan Recreation Passport required

out, and spaced so that you tend to forget the neighbors altogether. At each end, sites 2–4 and 22 and 23, the sandy rise goes to ground and campers enjoy a less obstructed view of the distant lake. These are the ones to pick if you like that morning sunrise coming up over the water.

With the exception of 7, the only site to fall on the west side of the road, trails lead from the individual campsites out to the water. The bay warms up nicely in the summer and is great for swimming.

At the north end of the campground, you will find the trailhead for the Ninga Aki Pathway. This 2.5-mile walk in the woods features 15 interpretive stations, describing different natural features and the role they played in the lives of the Ojibwa people. The first of the pathway's two loops takes you back to Bog Lake—portions of the trail follow a boardwalk over wetland. The other loop follows the

shore of Lake Michigan before curving back to the campground.

From its base just west of Manistique, the Garden Peninsula stretches south into Lake Michigan. On a regional map, it looks as if it is reaching out to touch the tip of Wisconsin's Door Peninsula. To the west, the peninsula defines Big Bay de Noc, the little sister to Green Bay. The peninsula is, in fact, part of the grand Niagara Escarpment, which stretches from upstate New York to Wisconsin.

On the opposite side of the peninsula, west and a little south, you will find one of the state's most interesting parks—Fayette Historic State Park. The campground at Fayette is comfortable enough. RVs and trailers have room to spare, but the site isn't overdeveloped. Described as semimodern, the campground has vault toilets, hand-pumped water, and electrical service.

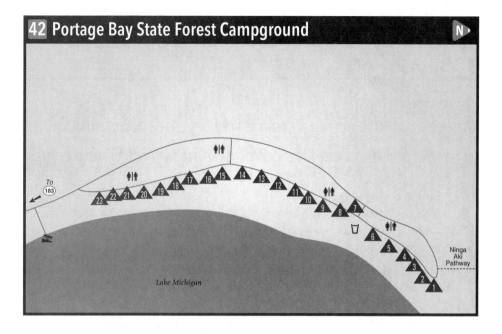

42 Portage Bay State Forest Campground

Most visitors come to the park to roam through the Fayette Historic Townsite. In the late 1880s, this collection of old buildings was once a bustling company town. The Jackson Iron Company took iron ore and turned it into pig iron to be shipped to plants making steel. The town sits along a natural harbor, partly hemmed in by a long dolomite cliff. The old furnace complex overlooks the water.

Visitors tend to be surprised by how much of the old town is actually left. You can still visit the Shelton Hotel, the old town hall, the machine shop, and the company office. Out on the wooded point that outlines the other side of the harbor, homes of the doctor and company superintendent remain for you to visit. Throughout the summer, boats pull into Snail Shell Harbor and tie up at the dock.

:: Getting There

From Manistique, follow US 2 west 16 miles to M 183. Turn south and drive 20 miles. You will pass through the village of Garden. As you approach the turn for LL Road, M 183 makes a 90-degree turn west (this is the second such turn; the first is just south of Garden). LL Road continues south. Less than 1.5 miles down, turn east on 12.75 Lane. You should see signs. The campground is at the end of this road, 5 winding miles to the east.

GPS COORDINATES   N45° 43.434'   W86° 32.106'

43

Carney Lake State Forest Campground

Rather than distracting from the scenery, the cabins give the place the feel of an old North Woods hunting and fishing camp.

As you head west across the Upper Peninsula, Dickinson County is the first you come to that doesn't touch either Lake Michigan or Lake Superior. Only two counties in the Upper Peninsula can be called landlocked, and the other is Dickinson's neighbor to the west, Iron County. Here, the boundaries are defined not by the glacial basins of the Great Lakes but by the meandering paths of the Brule and Menominee Rivers. US 2, the main east–west highway, cuts across from Escanaba, turning northwest in Iron Mountain, and continues into Wisconsin for a spell before reaching Crystal Falls and eventually Ironwood.

Northeast of Iron Mountain—far from where the Porcupine Mountains overlook the cold gray of Lake Superior

:: Ratings

BEAUTY: ★ ★ ★ ★
PRIVACY: ★ ★ ★ ★
SPACIOUSNESS: ★ ★ ★ ★ ★
QUIET: ★ ★ ★ ★ ★
SECURITY: ★ ★ ★ ★ ★
CLEANLINESS: ★ ★ ★ ★

and hours from the sandy dune beaches of Lake Michigan—you will find a really nice place to camp, though it takes some driving. First, you drive north to Merriman and then head east along Forest Service roads. Six miles of gravel roller coaster later, Carney Lake waits in a forest of white pines and birches. You will find the campground at the northwest corner of the lake.

Carney Lake State Forest Campground consists of a simple loop of 16 grassy campsites. You can't make reservations here, so you obviously can't always count on getting the exact site you want, but the campground sees light use throughout the summer, and a happy alternative site is almost always available. Six sites along the lake have trails leading down to the water. Site 9 sits on a rise with a great view of Carney Lake. More graveled and open than the rest, this site, I imagine, is popular for campers towing a small trailer.

The facilities are limited to vault toilets and water from a hand pump; however, on my last visit a sign indicated that bacteria levels in the well had reached an unsafe level, and the well was locked. I am not sure how the problem is being

:: Key Information

ADDRESS: 1933 US 2, Crystal Falls, MI 49920

OPERATED BY: Michigan DNR– Bewabic State Park

CONTACT: 906-875-3324; tinyurl.com/3ab2gd2

OPEN: Year-round, though snow will prevent access in winter

SITES: 16

EACH SITE: Picnic table and fire pit

ASSIGNMENT: First come, first served

REGISTRATION: Self-register at campground.

FACILITIES: Hand-pumped potable water and vault toilets

PARKING: At site

FEE: $13

ELEVATION: 1,129 feet

RESTRICTIONS:

■ **Pets:** On leash only

■ **Fires:** Fire pits only

■ **Vehicles:** 2 per site; Michigan Recreation Passport required

addressed, so I'd bring a container of water, just in case. The closest water supply would be at the Summer Breeze Campground, just a few miles south of Sportsmens Club Road off of M 95, if they're amenable. This private campground is more suitable to RVs, but in addition to water, it has a great camp store.

Carney Lake itself is a gem. Surrounded by woods, a few cabins on the far shore are set back into the trees. Rather than distracting from the scenery, they add to it, giving the place that feel of an old North Woods hunting and fishing camp. The lake reaches 30 feet deep out in front of the campground, and the southwest half of the lake is a much shallower 10–20 feet. All told, its surface area spreads out over 117 acres.

Bring your boat and cast a line for smallmouth bass, walleye, northern pike, pumpkinseed, and sunfish. The lake drains to the north, and at both ends you will find marsh and swampland. Rocks and gravel, however, line both the campground side of the lake and the opposite shore.

Part of the campground's appeal is how little else there is to do here but camp (and perhaps fish). For more recreational-type activities, consider a trip south to the 1,800-acre Fumee Lake Natural Area, due east of Iron Mountain. You will have to drive back through town and access the park from US 2. Four main trails offer everything from easygoing 1.5-mile hikes to strenuous 4.4-mile loops. An additional 4.5 miles of rugged single-track are open to hikers, mountain bikers, and, in the winter, cross-country skiers. The centerpiece of the preserve is the 507-acre Fumee Lake, which, combined with neighboring Little Fumee, offers 5 miles of undeveloped shoreline. The area is used by educators to teach ecology and

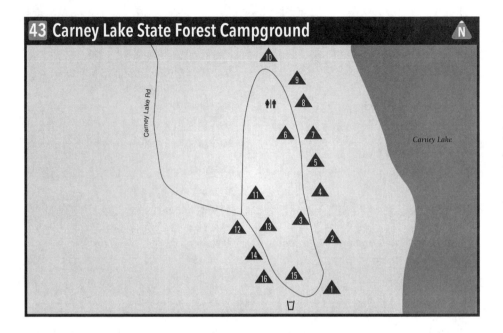

43 Carney Lake State Forest Campground

is home to common loons, bald eagles, and 17 different species of orchids.

At some point, stop by Damian's Pasta Works in Iron Mountain for some of the best Italian food in the state. European immigrants poured into the Upper Peninsula in the 19th century, looking for work in the mines. Throughout the UP, communities still reflect the influence of their old-world forebears, many of whom came from such places as Norway, Finland, Italy, and England and usually settled in enclaves with their own people. The Italian restaurants here are legendary. Damian's does away with the usual amenities (such as tables and chairs) and best suits the camping ethos. The menu has the usual Italian fare with some local additions. Order from the counter and take away boxes of linguine, fettuccine, or good old spaghetti with one of their 10 sauces. They also have pastries and excellent sandwiches.

:: Getting There

Driving about 7.5 miles north of Iron Mountain on M 95, you will come to the tiny community of Merriman—no more than a couple of shops on the corner, all of which looked out of business during my last visit. Turn right here on Sportsmens Club Road. After 2.6 miles, you come to a T at Carney Lake Road. Turn right, following Carney Lake Road 4 miles back to the campground on the lake.

GPS COORDINATES   N45° 53.526'   W87° 56.496'

44

Bewabic State Park Campground

The terrain throughout the park is hilly and wooded, and the ground behind many sites falls away into a forest of pines and maples.

Crossing **US 2** from Iron Mountain to Crystal Falls, dipping into Wisconsin along the way, you are passing through the Upper Peninsula's Menominee Range. Iron mining was a booming industry here not too long ago, and you see evidence of this everywhere you go in this part of the state. The Ojibwa word for iron was pewabic. The presence of this metal in the Upper Peninsula was known for centuries, and throughout the Upper Peninsula you will find this word, and its many variations, tacked to a lot of different things—Pewabick Falls on the Little Iron River; the community of Pewabic on the Keweenaw Peninsula; and here, just north of the

:: Ratings

BEAUTY: ★ ★ ★ ★ ★
PRIVACY: ★ ★ ★ ★ ★
SPACIOUSNESS: ★ ★ ★ ★ ★
QUIET: ★ ★ ★ ★
SECURITY: ★ ★ ★ ★ ★
CLEANLINESS: ★ ★ ★ ★ ★

Wisconsin border, Bewabic State Park. (You find the same word spelled so many different ways because each person who came to learn the native languages wrote the sounds they heard differently. Bishop Baraga wrote *biwabic*, whereas early French explorers wrote it as *piouabic*.)

Bewabic State Park is 4 miles west of Crystal Falls, right off US 2. This 315-acre park features a large campground with modern and semimodern sites, tennis courts (a state-park rarity), a beach and bathhouse on the Fortune Lakes, and a short nature trail. Two sets of modern restrooms have running water and flush toilets, and the bathhouse in the day-use area has showers. Though fully prepared to host a troop of RVs, the campground is rather tent-friendly.

The 137 sites that make up the campground, which is well used throughout the season and is very shaded, are organized around three loops. The first loop, with sites 1–28, offers perhaps the best spots for tent camping in the park (I'll

:: Key Information

ADDRESS: 1933 US 2, Crystal Falls, MI 49920

OPERATED BY: Michigan DNR–Bewabic State Park

CONTACT: 906-875-3324; **michigan.gov/bewabic**

OPEN: Mid-May–November 1

SITES: 137

EACH SITE: Picnic table and fire pit; some have power.

ASSIGNMENT: First come, first served during off-season; during peak season, reservations can be made online at **midnrreservations.com** and by calling 800-447-2757.

REGISTRATION: Register at campground office.

FACILITIES: Beach house with flushable toilets, bathhouse, and 4 vault toilets

PARKING: At site

FEE: Walk-in sites $16 ($10 off-season); others $20 ($16 off-season)

ELEVATION: 1,407 feet

RESTRICTIONS:

■ **Pets:** On leash only (maximum 6 feet); no pets on beach

■ **Fires:** Fire pits or grills only

■ **Vehicles:** Permit required; only 2 per site; additional vehicles can be parked by campground office.

mention one notable exception later when looking at the third loop). The sites around this loop lie on the outside of the circle, facing in toward the wooded center. The terrain throughout the park is hilly and wooded, and the ground behind many sites falls away into a forest of pines and maples. Though officially part of the modern campground, none of the sites here have electrical hookups, there are no pull-through sites, and the dedicated bathroom facility is a pit toilet. The smattering of grass that covers the lots has a rough go of it, and campers are as likely to find a grassy spot as one of packed dirt on which to pitch a tent.

Sites 29–81 on the second loop have decent lots against the loop's eastern side.

Stick with sites 57–73, and you should do okay. Sites at the front of the loop, close to the modern restrooms, have electrical hookups and attract a different kind of camper.

The third loop includes sites 82–137 and has a strange mix of sites. Here, most of the lots come with electricity. Against the back are 11 pull-through sites. If RVs and fifth-wheels are to be found anywhere in the campground, it is here. That said, at the south end of the drive is a parking area for the park's four walk-in campsites. These are the exception I mentioned before. Decent buffers between sites throughout the campground provide ample privacy, but that doesn't compare with having your own spot in the woods.

Located in a grove of tall maples, these walk-in sites each have a picnic table and fire pit, as well as a raised tent pad. The rolling forest floor makes this last item a necessity. The silence of the woods at these sites is broken only by the sound of the wind in the trees high above and the echo of twigs and sap falling on the blanket of last year's leaves below.

The state park is located on the northernmost of the Fortune Lakes. This chain of four lakes—aptly named First Lake, Second Lake, and so on—is popular with anglers who catch perch, walleye, pike, and bass. The lakes are connected by small channels and give paddlers some interesting water for exploring. First Lake also connects to Mud Lake, north of US 2.

First Lake is the largest of the bunch, and the park covers nearly the entire western shore, most of it undeveloped. The day-use area features a picnic shelter, a playground, tennis courts, a bathhouse, and a fine swimming beach. You will immediately notice the stone pavilion, which was built by the Civilian Conservation Corps in the 1930s. From the beach a trail heads east to a footbridge that leads to a small island.

Beyond the park are a number of sites that highlight the region's mining history. Close by is Fortune Pond, just a half mile north of US 2 on North Bristol Road, halfway between the park and Crystal Falls. The small lake here was once an open-pit iron mine that, in the 1950s, cranked out well more than a million tons of iron ore. The county maintains a small park on the east side of the pond. The clear, deep water has attracted scuba divers by the score. At the end of the fishing pier, the bottom of the lake drops to 35 feet, and you can see all the way down. This is just one of the stops on the Iron County Heritage Trail (**ironheritage.org**), which connects historic sites from Crystal Falls to Iron River. To get a sense of the contribution iron mining has made to the region, be sure to stop at a few of these sites while you're in the area.

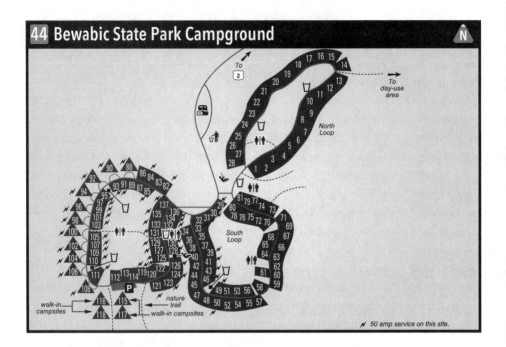

:: Getting There

From downtown Crystal Falls, where US 2 and US 141 enter town from the south, follow US 2 for 4.5 miles west to the state park.

GPS COORDINATES N46° 05.658' W88° 25.524'

45

Sylvania Wilderness and Recreation Area:
CLARK LAKE CAMPGROUND

Clark Lake is just the beginning when it comes to camping in the Sylvania Wilderness.

The **Ottawa National Forest** manages nearly a million acres in Michigan's western Upper Peninsula, and perhaps none of it is as ruggedly beautiful as the 18,327 acres set aside as the Sylvania Wilderness and Recreation Area (SWRA). In the late 1800s, a lumberman from Wisconsin purchased 80 acres south of Clark Lake, which is several miles southwest of Watersmeet. He was so impressed with the magnificence of the region that he decided to keep the property as a private preserve. He soon introduced others to this primeval forest, and they too snatched up acreage. They soon established the Sylvan Club and built lodges and cabins to better enjoy

:: Ratings

BEAUTY: ★ ★ ★ ★ ★
PRIVACY: ★ ★ ★ ★
SPACIOUSNESS: ★ ★ ★ ★ ★
QUIET: ★ ★ ★ ★
SECURITY: ★ ★ ★ ★ ★
CLEANLINESS: ★ ★ ★ ★ ★

their rustic playground. In 1967, the U.S. Forest Service purchased the land; 20 years later, the land joined several other tracts recognized by the Michigan Wilderness Act.

Most of the forest in the Upper Peninsula, and the Lower Peninsula for that matter, was harvested in the late 19th and early 20th centuries. What you see today, even in the most remote national and state forests, is second growth, woods less than a hundred years old. A few pockets of virgin stands here and there offer a glimpse of the old Michigan. The Sylvania Wilderness offers more than a glimpse. Here you can immerse yourself for a week of camping in an authentic North Country woods.

Not everyone has the resources and opportunity for backcountry adventure, so the Forest Service maintains a regular, semimodern campground near the entrance to the wilderness area. The Clark Lake Campground allows campers a chance to spend a few days walking or

:: Key Information

ADDRESS: County Road 535, Watersmeet, MI 49969

OPERATED BY: Ottawa National Forest, Watersmeet Ranger District

CONTACT: 906-358-4551; tinyurl.com/pth9o7r

OPEN: Late May–November

SITES: 48

EACH SITE: Picnic table, fire pit with grill, and lantern post

ASSIGNMENT: First come, first served

REGISTRATION: Self-register at campground; pay for permit at the Sylvania Entrance Station.

FACILITIES: Pressurized drinking water, flush and vault toilets, and modern restrooms

PARKING: At site

FEE: $14 for camping, plus $5 permit fee; annual permits $20

ELEVATION: 885 feet

RESTRICTIONS:

■ **Pets:** On leash only

■ **Fires:** Fire pits only

paddling into the Sylvania Tract without all the gear and preparation that comes with loading up a canoe for a week on the water.

The campground holds 48 sites on four loops. This is a national forest, after all, so it's no surprise to find the campground nestled in the woods, mostly pines interspersed with hardwoods. Campsite spurs are packed gravel, but the sites tend to be grassy. Throughout the camp you will find a nice mix—wooded lots with lots of privacy versus wide-open sites, spaces with room to spread out but also a few cozy nooks tucked into the trees. There's no need to recommend one loop over another; just find a site you like and stake your claim. In fact, because reservations are not an option at Clark Lake, that's exactly what you'll have to do.

The sites here feature the usual national-forest campground amenities— wooden picnic table, lantern post, and fire pit with an iron grill. Brick bathrooms with running hot water and flush toilets are spaced evenly throughout, and down by the day-use area you will find men's and women's shower rooms. I can't speak for the ladies, but the men's side is an open locker-room style shower. With its concrete-slab floors and cinder-block walls, this building has seen better days, but if you wait long enough, the water eventually warms a little, and that's enough of a luxury sometimes to overcome dingy surroundings.

Spend much time looking at a map of the Sylvania Tract (as some folks call it), and you will see that Clark Lake is just the beginning when it comes to camping in the Sylvania Wilderness. Another 50 sites are located throughout the park. (These you must reserve.) Most are only accessible by canoe, though there is a nice trail system that passes a number of the sites, and backpackers will use these from time to time.

Paddlers access the wilderness from one of two boat landings. Clark Lake has a parking area, with shower and restroom facilities and a boat launch. The lake has 11 backcountry sites along its shore, and this is the most popular put-in for paddlers heading into the park. The other landing can be found east of the campground along County Road 535. Crooked Lake also has a parking area, and the short trail leading from the parking lot to the boat launch is itself a scenic preview to what awaits visitors making their way into the wild. The waters here are relatively clear. You will find that many of the Upper Peninsula's lakes and rivers are stained brown by tannins (this is how the Black River and the Tahquamenon's Root Beer Falls get their names). The waters of Sylvania, on the other hand, are a clear blue-green.

The SWRA has often been called Michigan's answer to the Boundary Waters Canoe Area. While not nearly as expansive, with somewhat different geology (Boundary Waters tends to have rockier terrain), Sylvania does offer some of the same North Country charms you find in Minnesota. When planning a trip through the SWRA, campers have fewer options in regards to routes and distances, but once the packs are loaded (whether they are backpacks or Duluth packs) and the trip is underway, the sense of solitude is the same. There is still the soft ripple when a paddle touches the water, the sound of loons calling in the distance, and perhaps an eagle flying high above. And there's the same distance from civilization that campers crave.

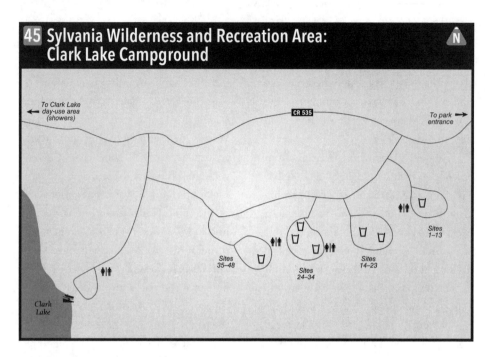

:: Getting There

Almost exactly 4 miles west of Watersmeet on US 2, turn south on CR 535 (Thousand Island Lake Road). In 4 miles you will come to the Sylvania Entrance Station. It is here you can grab a map and pay for your permit. Continuing past the station, the road comes to a T. Turn left, and the campground is down a couple thousand feet on your left.

GPS COORDINATES   N46° 14.478'   W89° 19.248'

46

Bond Falls Flowage Campground

Once you visit Bond Falls, just north of the flowage, you will understand why so many people love this place.

There appears to always be some controversy circling the Bond Falls Flowage north of Watersmeet. The lake and most of the land around it belong to the Upper Peninsula Power Company (UPPCO). Power companies are never very popular with nature lovers in the first place, and when a company owns a piece of property as picturesque and naturally beautiful as this, and its policies in turn affect one of the Upper Peninsula's most popular waterfalls and the quality of the river downstream, there's sure to be a concerned outcry over every decision. In recent years the UPPCO sold off acreage around the lake for development (though the developer now wants out and has

taken the matter to court), expanded the campground, and rebuilt the dam leading to Bond Falls. Each of these decisions has, at the very least, been the cause of some discussion.

Interestingly, the immense 2,100-acre lake that many seem anxious to protect from the power company was created by the power company. It is the result of a dam built on the Middle Branch of the Ontonagon River back in 1937. Water from the river and several feeder streams is captured in this reservoir and diverted by way of a flume to the South Branch of the Ontonagon River. The lake provides water to the Victoria Reservoir farther north, which requires a steady supply to power its generators. The flowage itself is a happy accident of the company's harnessing of the river to provide electricity to Copper Country.

Once you visit Bond Falls, just north of the flowage, you will understand why so many people love this place. It's a beautiful spot in the woods, and there is a lot to do and see. The region includes

:: Ratings

BEAUTY: ★ ★ ★ ★ ★
PRIVACY: ★ ★ ★ ★ ★
SPACIOUSNESS: ★ ★ ★ ★ ★
QUIET: ★ ★ ★ ★ ★
SECURITY: ★ ★ ★ ★
CLEANLINESS: ★ ★ ★ ★

:: Key Information

ADDRESS: UPPCO Hydro Office, P.O. Box 357, Ishpeming, MI 49849

OPERATED BY: Upper Peninsula Power Company

CONTACT: 906-827-3753; **uppco.com /company/pdf/bondfalls.pdf**

OPEN: June–September 15

SITES: 48

EACH SITE: Picnic table, fire pit with grill, and lantern post

ASSIGNMENT: First come, first served

REGISTRATION: Register at Bond Falls Outpost.

FACILITIES: Hand-pumped water and vault toilets

PARKING: At site

FEE: $8

ELEVATION: 1,439 feet

RESTRICTIONS:

■ **Pets:** On leash only

■ **Fires:** In grills, fireplace, or fire pits only

■ **Vehicles:** 2 per site

the Bond Falls Scenic Area, a day-use area on the north shore of the lake, and a fine campground of 48 sites spread out like a necklace around much of the lake. The campsites here can be divided into two groups. The first consists of the 20 sites found in the Bond Falls Consolidated Campground on the western shore of the lake. Located on a small point, paths to the west, north, and east lead to the water. Tucked into woods as they are, even this, the largest grouping of sites on the lake, offers a decent amount of privacy. There are several pull-through sites, and the facilities are accessible to folks using wheelchairs.

The dispersed sites around the flowage can be found along the west, north, and east shores. Bond Falls Road follows the lake around its west and north shores, and the campsites here are the easiest to

get to. The choicest of the lot are those to the east—sites E1–E16. Sites E5–E7 sit at the base of a long point and face the setting sun, a nice feature anytime, but early and late in the season this means a longer evening in camp. Facilities throughout include vault toilets and water from hand pumps. Each site features a fire pit with grill and picnic table. Campers often bring their canoes and simply launch from the shore.

As spectacular as this lake is, most visitors come to Bond Falls for the waterfall. Considered by many to be the most stunning falls in the Upper Peninsula, the river here tumbles 50 feet down a pyramid of boulders and rock. At its base, the water collects in a large pool before continuing south. A narrow trail leads up the rocks on the west side of the river, and you can get a great view this way. The state runs the Bond Falls Scenic Area, and a vehicle permit is required to park here. But come from camp or Bond Falls Road, and a nice trail leads to the upper side of the falls. Around its base a wide, somewhat ornate boardwalk keeps your feet dry and allows you to see the cascade from a number of perspectives.

Downstream, near M 28, the Ontonagon takes another tumble, this time a 40-foot drop down Agate Falls—certainly worth a visit. The water from Bond Falls to the confluence of the various Ontonagons north of here can be a little shallow, but, upstream, the Middle Branch can be navigated by canoe as far south

as Watersmeet. From the bridge at US 45 to the flowage, you will find more than 20 miles of good water. There are a few portages in there, so be sure to check out a decent river guide. The whole journey could take up to 10 hours, and a lot of folks choose to camp about halfway at the Ottawa National Forest's Burneda Dam Campground.

Boat launches are located on both the north and south ends of the lake. And at the dam above the falls, the kids will love stopping for some ice cream or other concessions at the Bond Falls Outpost. The store also sells souvenirs and some camp supplies.

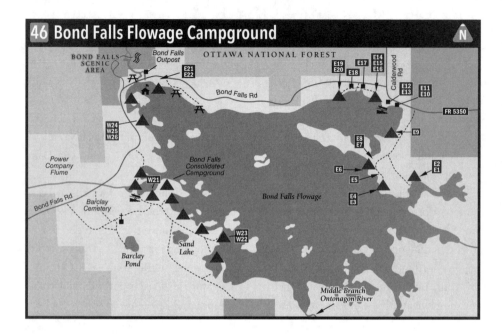

:: Getting There

Drive north of Watersmeet on US 45 for 9.5 miles to Bond Falls Road. Take the road east 3 miles to the Bond Falls Outpost. There, you can find a map of the campground and register.

GPS COORDINATES N46° 24.492' W89° 07.800'

47

Henry Lake National Forest Campground

Carved out of a mix of hardwoods and pines, the campsites are spacious and grassy, and many are edged in thick ferns.

You will find four campgrounds in this book from the western Upper Peninsula's Gogebic County—that is twice what any other county can boast. Henry Lake is probably the most humble of the bunch. Both Black River Harbor and the Presque Isle Campground in the Porcupine Mountains State Wilderness front Lake Superior. Clark Lake serves as a doorway to the legendary Sylvania Wilderness. Henry Lake, on the other hand, offers 11 quiet sites on a small lake. The farthest west of a series of national-forest campgrounds that lie between US 2 and the Wisconsin border, Henry Lake is representative of the region's camping.

:: Ratings

BEAUTY: ★ ★ ★ ★
PRIVACY: ★ ★ ★ ★ ★
SPACIOUSNESS: ★ ★ ★ ★ ★
QUIET: ★ ★ ★ ★ ★
SECURITY: ★ ★ ★ ★ ★
CLEANLINESS: ★ ★ ★ ★ ★

Neighboring campgrounds include Moosehead Lake, Pomeroy Lake, Bobcat Lake, and Langford Lake.

The pattern you notice here tells a lot about the local geography: There are many lakes just south of US 2 once you get west of Watersmeet. If you expand the region to include the area south into Wisconsin, you will find country over-flowing with hundreds of lakes. You also find an important watershed. Most of the lakes on the Michigan side of the bor-der flow into Lake Superior. Those south make their way to the Mississippi. (It's not until you get a bit farther east that the lakes and streams of northern Wisconsin begin to flow toward Lake Michigan.)

In the heart of a national forest, lakes and rivers, and camping facilities, you find the 43-acre Henry Lake and its truly hospitable campground. Eleven grassy sites line up along the north shore of the lake. Most are too far back for a view of the water, but three of them—sites 5, 7, and 9—let you see the lake from camp. Carved out of a mix of hardwoods and pines, the

:: Key Information

ADDRESS: 500 North Moore Street, Bessemer, MI 49911

OPERATED BY: Ottawa National Forest, Bessemer Ranger District

CONTACT: 906-932-1330; tinyurl.com/l3qwx9f

OPEN: Mid-May–mid-September

SITES: 11

EACH SITE: Picnic table and fire pit

ASSIGNMENT: First come, first served

REGISTRATION: Register at the entrance pay station.

FACILITIES: Hand-pumped water and vault toilets

PARKING: At site

FEE: $12

ELEVATION: 1,592 feet

RESTRICTIONS:

■ **Pets:** On leash only

■ **Fires:** Fire pits only

campsites are spacious and grassy, and many are edged in thick ferns. The sites themselves are set far back from the road and offer all the privacy in the world.

Two vault toilets near the campground entrance and one at the boat launch, as well as water from a hand pump, complete the camp's list of luxuries. A boat launch and a fishing pier round out the facilities. Located this far north and quite a drive from the closest town, the campground feels safe, even without a host camper overseeing the property.

Henry Lake is relatively shallow, only 30 feet deep at the middle. Fish attractors at the fishing pier and directly across the lake from the pier provide habitat and help support the fishery of largemouth

bass, bluegills, perch, and pumpkinseed (a sunfish so named for its unique coloring). The lake has a wide gravel boat ramp, and the pier east of the ramp is accessible by wheelchair. A nice packed-gravel trail leads from the parking area out to the dock.

The West Branch of the Presque Isle River flows close to Lake Henry. The upper portions of the Presque Isle offer easy paddling, suitable for newbies. Farther downstream, however, the Presque Isle serves up some of the most dangerous, yet at times still doable, whitewater in the state. For the easy stretch of river, put in at the Teal canoe landing north of Henry Lake on Forest Road 8100. This puts you on the West Branch of the river. The trip will take you through the Presque Isle River Flooding and north of US 2. At one point, there's a long portage around Yondata Falls. After that, the river continues at a leisurely pace to M 28. Canoeing or kayaking north of M 28 is for experts, and even they sometimes balk at the challenge.

Taking advantage of miles of Forest Service roads, the Pomeroy/Henry Lake Mountain Bike Complex offers mountain bikers 100 miles of loops through the national forest and around numerous lakes. This isn't the kind of mountain biking that sends you flying through the woods down steep singletrack, braking and leaning hard into the turns, or hopping over downed logs. This is the place, rather, where the whole family can ride together. You don't really even need a mountain bike to tackle these loops, which have an easy grade and moderate hills, though folks with thin-tired road bikes will run into some trouble. To get a map of all the loops, stop by the Western Upper Peninsula Convention & Visitor Bureau in Ironwood, or give them a call at 906-932-4850.

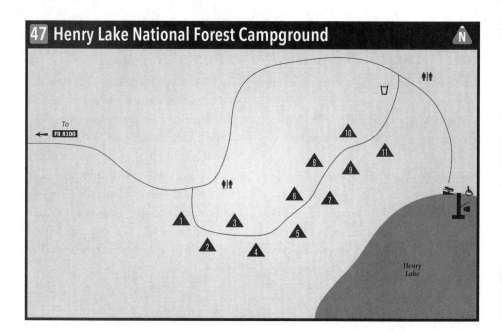

:: Getting There

From US 2, follow M 64 south into and through the town of Marenisco. Continue south 5.6 miles to FR 8100. Turn right (west). The campground is 4.6 miles in.

GPS COORDINATES   N46° 19.824'   W89° 47.556'

Black River Harbor National Forest Campground

Campers looking for a little recreation can use the North Country Trail as an out-and-back that will take them by all the significant falls on the Black River.

You will find scenic waterfalls throughout the Upper Peninsula. And while the eastern Upper Peninsula has Tahquamenon, Miners Falls, and perhaps Laughing Whitefish (the latter depending on where you draw the boundary between east and west), travelers making a waterfall tour don't really hit their stride until they get west of Marquette. With a decent waterfall map in hand, you will pass close by some cataract or other, whatever route you take. There you have beauties, such as Black River Falls and Canyon Falls. Farther west are Bond Falls, north of Watersmeet, and

:: Ratings

BEAUTY: ★ ★ ★ ★ ★
PRIVACY: ★ ★ ★ ★
SPACIOUSNESS: ★ ★ ★ ★ ★
QUIET: ★ ★ ★ ★
SECURITY: ★ ★ ★ ★ ★
CLEANLINESS: ★ ★ ★ ★ ★

Agate Falls, downriver from that, near M 28. An important route to add to any waterfall-viewing itinerary is the Black River Harbor Parkway (also known as Black River Road).

For 11 miles the road parallels the Black River, ending at Black River Harbor. In 1992, it was designated a National Forest Scenic Byway. The drive alone—winding and thickly wooded—would be worth the trip, but the real attractions along the byway are a series of five waterfalls and the day-use area at the journey's end.

It is here, right before the harbor, that the national forest has established the Black River Harbor Campground. Forty sites are situated on one large loop, tucked in between maple and birch trees. The camp offers water from a spigot and two sets of restrooms with flush toilets. The bathrooms can be found inside the loop at either end, quite set apart from the campsites. As you drive the paved road through the campground, you'll notice wide mowed paths, always on your

:: Key Information

<table>
<tr>
<td>

ADDRESS: 500 North Moore Street, Bessemer, MI 49911

OPERATED BY: Ottawa National Forest, Bessemer Ranger District

CONTACT: 906-932-1330; tinyurl.com/ldecw3b

OPEN: Late May–September

SITES: 40

EACH SITE: Picnic table and fire pit

ASSIGNMENT: First come, first served

REGISTRATION: Self-register at campground.

</td>
<td>

FACILITIES: Pressurized water and toilets

PARKING: At site

FEE: $16

ELEVATION: 738 feet

RESTRICTIONS:

■ **Pets:** On leash only

■ **Fires:** Fire pits only

■ **Vehicles:** 2 per site

</td>
</tr>
</table>

left. Once inside the circle, all these pathways eventually lead to the toilets. There are no showers here.

Sites are spacious and grassy and come with a picnic table and fire pit. (There are more picnic tables overlooking Lake Superior and in the day-use area.) None of the campsites have a view of Lake Superior; though, at the northern end of camp, the Great Lake is just through the trees. A path leads down to the water and a wide sandy beach.

This tends to be a busy campground throughout summer. Registration is on a first-come, first-serve basis. The next closest campground is to the east in the Porcupines Mountain Wilderness Area. Less than 5 miles away if you were to walk the shore of Lake Superior, Presque Isle Campground (see page 195) will take you more than an hour—38 miles, all told—to reach by car. Other nearby campgrounds

include Little Girl's Point (operated by Gogebic County), which is northwest of Ironwood on the lake; the other rustic and modern campgrounds in the Porcupine Mountains; and the national forest facilities southeast of Ironwood.

Waterfall hunters should look out for four trailheads along the Black River Harbor Parkway. These paths lead to five waterfalls: Great Conglomerate Falls, Potawatomi Falls, Gorge Falls, Sandstone Falls, and Rainbow Falls (in order, south to north). Three other named falls are upstream: Narrows, Chippewa Falls, and Algonquin Falls. These are less impressive (Narrows doesn't even merit the word falls in its name) and harder to get to.

Potawatomi Falls and Gorge Falls share a trailhead, and, if you only have time for one stop, make it this one. Potawatomi drops 30 feet in a gentle cascade. In low water, the falls divide around the large rock. The Gorge Falls downstream are no less impressive—dropping 25 feet through dark canyon walls.

One way to visit the falls is to hike awhile on the North Country Trail. The NCT enters the area from the east, just south of Rainbow Falls. It follows the river north to the harbor and then doubles back on the west side of the river. The pathway leaves Lake Superior here, heading inland, and unless thru-hikers add the optional Superior Hiking Trail in northern Minnesota, they will not draw as close to the Great Lakes again. Campers looking for a little recreation can use the trail as an out-and-back that will take them by all the significant falls on the Black River.

The NCT crosses the Black River over a suspension bridge close to the harbor. On either side of the river's mouth, sandy beach stretches in both directions. The bridge gets you over the river to enjoy the eastern portion of the day-use area. Black River Recreation Area One is one of only two harbors in the national-forest system.

The park features restrooms, a small store selling concessions and supplies for boaters, and a nice place to picnic under the pines and hemlocks.

In the fall, late September and early October, the trees in this part of the country seem to catch on fire. Brilliant reds and oranges draw fall-color tourists from all over. One of the best views of this autumnal transformation can be found at the south end of the scenic byway at the Copper Peak Ski Flying Hill (the only place in the Western Hemisphere where skiers can practice this extreme version of ski jumping). During the off-season, Copper Peak offers its Adventure Ride. First, the chairlift takes visitors 360 feet up to the top of Copper Peak (so named because copper is in the rocks). Then, an elevator takes them up another 18 stories (180 feet) to the top of the ski jump. On a good day, you can see Michigan, Wisconsin, Minnesota, and even Canada from this dizzying height. The view of the surrounding forest and Lake Superior is spectacular.

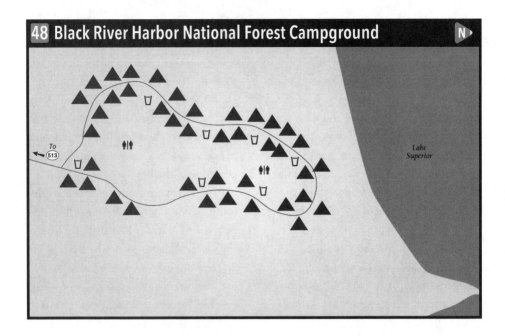

:: Getting There

From downtown Bessemer, drive 1.5 miles west on US 2 to Powderhorn Road (County Highway 511). After 3 miles, the road comes to a T at Black River Harbor Parkway (County Highway 513). Turn left and continue 11 miles to the campground entrance. If you miss it, the road ends a half mile later at Lake Superior and the Black River Harbor.

GPS COORDINATES   N46° 39.750'   W90° 03.120'

49

Porcupine Mountains Wilderness State Park:

PRESQUE ISLE CAMPGROUND

The wilderness area preserves the largest virgin stand of northern hardwoods west of the Adirondacks.

From a distance, these humped mountains along the southern shore of Lake Superior, bristling with old-growth northern hardwoods, are said to resemble a crouching porcupine. Henry Schoolcraft, a prodigious 19th-century explorer of the Northwest Territory, recorded the Chippewa name for the range as Kaug Wudju, their name for the prickly animal. Today, most people just call them the Porkies. As part of the 59,000-acre Porcupine Mountains Wilderness State Park, the mountains are the backdrop to some of the state's most stunning country. Rising up from

the Great Lake to well over a thousand feet, the mountains are lined with hard-worn hiking trails, veined with rivers and streams, and dotted with lakes—including the picturesque Lake of the Clouds.

The wilderness area preserves the largest virgin stand of northern hard-woods west of the Adirondacks. The character this lends to the Porkies is something you can't find elsewhere, and it attracts people from all over who have a lot of options when it comes to deciding how to take in the mountains. For many folks, the Porkies are a day trip. They drive up to the Lake of the Clouds overlook, take a few photos, and continue on their way. Others bring an RV or trailer and set up at the park's modern campground on Union Bay. Near the east entrance, Union Bay is the most popular spot to camp in the Porcupine Mountains. Still others strap on a backpack and head into the backcountry—whether they rent a remote cabin or yurt, or pitch a tent at one of the numerous backpack campsites

:: Ratings

BEAUTY: ★ ★ ★ ★ ★
PRIVACY: ★ ★ ★ ★
SPACIOUSNESS: ★ ★ ★ ★ ★
QUIET: ★ ★ ★ ★
SECURITY: ★ ★ ★ ★ ★
CLEANLINESS: ★ ★ ★ ★ ★

:: Key Information

ADDRESS: 33303 Headquarters Road, Ontonagon, MI 49953	**REGISTRATION:** Register at campground office.
OPERATED BY: Michigan DNR–Porcupine Mountains Wilderness State Park	**FACILITIES:** Water and vault toilets
	PARKING: At site
CONTACT: 906-885-5275; **michigan.gov/porkies**	**FEE:** $14
	ELEVATION: 695 feet
OPEN: Late April–late November	**RESTRICTIONS:**
SITES: 50	■ **Pets:** On leash only
EACH SITE: Picnic table and fire pit	■ **Fires:** Fire pits only
ASSIGNMENT: Reservations can be made online at **midnrreservations.com** or by calling 800-447-2757.	■ **Vehicles:** Michigan Recreation Passport required

along the trails, they see more than most visitors of this expansive wilderness.

At the western edge of the park, close to the waterfalls of Presque Isle River, the park service maintains a large rustic campground. Presque Isle Campground features 50 spacious sites on a lightly wooded bluff overlooking Lake Superior. Generators are allowed only at sites 28–42. That leaves 35 places to pitch your tent with a reasonable assurance of a quiet night. Along the generator side, against the east end of the loop, you'll find a couple of nice sites. Both 34 and 36 are set back among the towering hemlocks, white pines, and maples.

Sites along the northern edge of the campground look down from some height over Lake Superior, but they pay for this view with a lack of privacy from

neighboring campers. The choicest spots are at the western end of the main campground. Tent campers can access six walk-in sites by way of a narrow trail into the woods.

The amenities at Presque Isle are spare—vault toilets and water from a hand pump fill the list. There is, however, much to recommend the campground over Union Bay or the two smaller rustic sites located along South Boundary Road. From my perspective, the river makes all the difference. As the Presque Isle River finishes out its journey to Lake Superior, it puts on a final show, dropping 100 feet over its last mile. This results in three or four stunning waterfalls.

From the picnic area at the campground, you can cross the river near its mouth over a swinging bridge. Upstream from the bridge, you can see an unnamed falls. A boardwalk leads from the picnic area south along the west side of the river. Hike up the trail for views of Manabezho Falls, Manido Falls, and Nawadaha Falls (a side trail here leads down to the river for a better look). Once you get to South Boundary Road, cross the bridge and make the return trip on the east side of the river.

As you watch gallons of water pound their way down to Lake Superior, it might surprise you that there are people who paddle this river. Only very experienced whitewater kayakers and canoers will take on the challenge of the lower portions of the Presque Isle River, and even they will portage around many of the falls and rapids—including "the gorge," a stretch of whitewater where the river drops a stunning 140 feet in a mile.

There are a few things not to miss when visiting the Porkies. The Presque Isle waterfalls are just one. The other might just be the most photographed landscape in the state (maybe Michigan's answer to Colorado's Maroon Bells?). That would be the Lake of the Clouds. Located at some elevation behind the first big ridge along Lake Superior, the

Lake of the Clouds is stunningly beautiful. Most visitors drive up to the overlook and take in the scenery from the park's viewing platforms. During our last visit, a ranger kindly loaned us her binoculars and pointed out an eagle's nest in the valley below. If that peak doesn't satisfy, consider a hike on the Escarpment Trail.

The Porkies offer miles of hiking paths. The North Country Trail winds through the park, piggybacking on the system established by hikers long ago. The trails from the Presque Isle Campground lead you south along the river for a tour of the waterfalls. Others climb Summit Peak, the highest point in the park. One of the most stunning hikes in the Porcupine Mountains, perhaps in the state, follows the Escarpment Trail and offers breathtaking views of the Lake of the Clouds. The path can turn into a pretty strenuous 8-mile out-and-back, so be sure to know your limitations and check out a park map for ways to cut the trip short.

You will find maps at the Wilderness Visitor Center, which also has information on the park, including its various recreational opportunities.

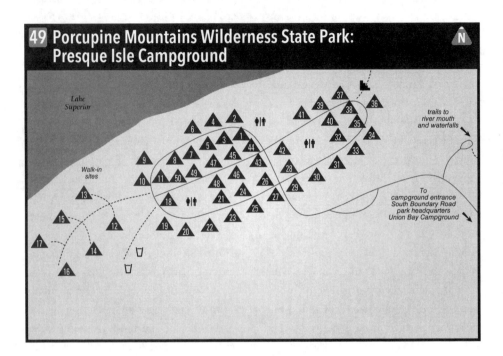

:: Getting There

From M 28 just northeast of Wakefield, turn north onto Presque Isle Road (County Road 519). Continue north 16.5 miles to the campground.

GPS COORDINATES   N46° 42.366'   W89° 58.716'

50

Courtney Lake National Forest Campground

A small inlet off Courtney Lake creates a point on which the two best sites in camp can be found.

This close to the Keweenaw Peninsula, you've officially entered the Upper Peninsula's Copper Country. The history of copper runs deep in this part of the world. The first explorers came here and heard of copper boulders too big for a man to carry. By that time, Native Americans had been pulling the pliable metal out of the ground for 7,000 years. It was widely traded—archaeologists find artifacts of Keweenaw copper throughout North America.

While most of the commercial mining during the 19th and 20th centuries took place on the peninsula proper, which is where you will find the Copper Country Trail National Scenic Byway,

such towns as nearby Mass City and Greenland once thrived on copper. Mass City mainly attracted immigrants from Finland—families who came a long way to eke a living out of the ground, both mining and farming where they could. Today, there are some reminders of the town's heyday, but you will see a lot of that gentle decay found in old mining towns all over the country.

Courtney Lake is about 8 miles east of Greenland and Mass City in the Ottawa National Forest. Located on this 33-acre lake is a small campground of 21 sites. On a low bluff covered in hardwoods, the campground wraps around the southwest corner of the lake, with beautifully situated sites overlooking the water. All of the sites feature a short packed-gravel spur for parking and grassy lots for pitching a tent. And in true national-forest fashion, they each come stocked with a picnic table, fire pit with an iron grill, and lantern post. Other facilities include vault toilets and water from a pressurized faucet.

:: Ratings

BEAUTY: ★ ★ ★ ★
PRIVACY: ★ ★ ★ ★
SPACIOUSNESS: ★ ★ ★ ★
QUIET: ★ ★ ★ ★ ★
SECURITY: ★ ★ ★ ★ ★
CLEANLINESS: ★ ★ ★ ★ ★

:: Key Information

ADDRESS: 1209 Rockland Drive, Ontonagon, MI 49953	**REGISTRATION:** Self-register at campground
OPERATED BY: Ottawa National Forest, Ontonagon Ranger District	**FACILITIES:** Pressurized water faucets and vault toilets
CONTACT: 906-884-2411; tinyurl.com/ldecw3b	**PARKING:** At site
OPEN: Late May–mid-October	**FEE:** $14
SITES: 21 (14 overlooking lake)	**ELEVATION:** 885 feet
EACH SITE: Picnic table, fire pit, and lantern post	**RESTRICTIONS:**
ASSIGNMENT: First come, first served	■ **Pets:** On leash only
	■ **Fires:** Fire pits only
	■ **Vehicles:** 2 per site

There's hardly an undesirable site to be found in the campground. Site 20 is particularly nice, as are 9 and 10. Site 9 offers less room than its neighbors but has a great view of the water. Site 10 sits back from the road, folded into a grove of surrounding pines. A small inlet off Courtney Lake creates a point on which the two best sites in camp can be found. Sites 15 and 16 are both walk-in sites, offering the most privacy and best access to the water. A sign designates these as being reserved for tent camping only—a message that seemed a little unnecessary given the posts blocking vehicles and trailers from progressing past the parking area.

Around camp, activities include boating and fishing on Courtney Lake, or swimming at the day-use area's small beach. A short 2.2-mile hike through the woods, complete with signage to annotate the trip, begins at a trailhead south of site 7. It is called the Circle of Life Interpretive Trail and includes a boardwalk platform for viewing a bog. Also nearby? The Old Grade Ski Trail. This old railroad grade, from a time when locomotives pulled lumber across the Upper Peninsula, has been repurposed as a cross-country-skiing trail. A nearly 2-mile path connects the campground to the main trail, which in turn offers 4.5 miles of skiing through the national forest. The path is groomed weekly during the season. Be aware, however, that the powers that be do not maintain the campground in the winter, and any snow that falls will remain until spring.

Beyond Courtney Lake, but not too far from the campground, the town of Greenland offers some short hikes with stunning views. On the hill above Greenland, you simply park at the Ontonagon County Fairgrounds. From there, a steep path continues up the hill. The first view you get is a look toward the northwest. From here, you can see all the way to Lake Superior. A little later on, the view to the southeast opens and you can see the forest spreading out to Mass City and beyond.

For an experience of the area's copper mining history and a diversion from the restful day-to-day of camp, visit the Adventure Copper Mine in Greenland. With hardhats and headlamps, visitors are led into the dark mine to learn firsthand the world of a miner. Though the mine was active for 70 years, beginning in 1850, you can still see copper in the walls. Bring a coat; it's chilly underground year-round. If the idea of the mine tour leaves you feeling claustrophobic, they also have surface tours and a decent little gift shop.

A bit of an aside: If your return trip takes you east along M 38 through L'Anse, be sure to stop at the Hilltop Restaurant and pick up one of their legendary cinnamon rolls. These gooey delights are huge and will leave you sticky and wanting more all the way home.

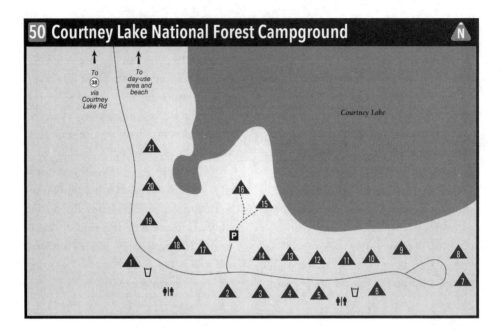

:: Getting There

The campground is about 8 miles east of Greenland (which is between Ontonagon and Baraga) on M 38. Courtney Lake Road leads south from the highway, and there's good signage all the way from M 38 a mile south to the campground.

GPS COORDINATES   N46° 45.096'   W88° 56.436'

APPENDIX A

● ●

Camping Equipment Checklist

Except for the large and bulky items on this list, I keep a plastic storage container full of the essentials for car camping so they're ready to go when I am. I make a last-minute check of the inventory, resupply anything that's low or missing, and away I go.

COOKING UTENSILS
Aluminum foil
Bottles of salt, pepper, spices, sugar,
    cooking oil, and maple syrup in
    waterproof, spillproof containers
Can and bottle openers
Cups, plastic or tin
Dish soap (biodegradable), sponge,
    towel
Flatware
Food of your choice
Frying pan
Fuel for stove
Lighter, matches in waterproof container
Plates
Pocketknife
Pot with lid
Spatula
Stove
Wooden spoon

FIRST-AID KIT
Adhesive bandages
Aspirin or ibuprofen
Diphenhydramine (Benadryl)
First-aid cream
Gauze pads
Insect repellent
Moleskin
Snakebite kit
Sunscreen and lip balm
Tape, waterproof adhesive

SLEEPING GEAR
Pillow
Sleeping bag
Sleeping pad, inflatable or insulated
Tent with ground tarp and rainfly

MISCELLANEOUS
Bath soap (biodegradable), washcloth,
    and towel
Camp chair
Candles
Cooler
Deck of cards
Fire starter
Flashlight with fresh batteries
Foul-weather clothing
GPS
Lantern
Maps (road, topographic, trails, etc.)
Paper towels
Plastic zip-top bags
Sunglasses
Toilet paper
Water bottle
Wool blanket

OPTIONAL
Barbecue grill
Binoculars
Field guides on bird, plant, and
    wildlife identification
Fishing rod and tackle
Hatchet

APPENDIX B

● ●

Sources of Information

ATLANTA FIELD OFFICE/
MACKINAW STATE FOREST
13501 M 33
Atlanta, MI 49709
989-785-4251

CADILLAC MANAGEMENT UNIT/
PERE MARQUETTE STATE FOREST
8015 Mackinaw Trail
Cadillac, MI 49601
231-775-9727

CRYSTAL FALLS FIELD OFFICE/
COPPER COUNTRY STATE FOREST
1420 US Highway 2
Crystal Falls, MI 49920
906-875-6622

GRAND TRAVERSE COUNTY
Parks and Recreation
1213 West Civic Center Drive
Traverse City, MI 49686
231-922-4818
co.grand-traverse.mi.us

GRAYLING FIELD OFFICE/
AU SABLE STATE FOREST
1955 Hartwick Pines Road
Grayling, MI 49738
989-732-3541

GWINN FIELD OFFICE/
ESCANABA RIVER STATE FOREST
410 West M 35
Gwinn, MI 49841
906-346-9201

HIAWATHA NATIONAL FOREST
2727 North Lincoln Road
Escanaba, MI 49829
906-786-4062
www.fs.usda.gov/hiawatha

HURON-MANISTEE NATIONAL
FOREST
Supervisors Office
1755 South Mitchell Street
Cadillac, MI 49601
800-821-6263
www.fs.usda.gov/hmnf

MICHIGAN DEPARTMENT OF
NATURAL RESOURCES
Recreation Division
Mason Building, Third Floor
P.O. Box 30031
Lansing, MI 48909
517-373-9900; **michigan.gov/dnr**

NEWBERRY FIELD OFFICE/
LAKE SUPERIOR STATE FOREST
Box 428
Newberry, MI 49868
906-293-3293

OTTAWA NATIONAL FOREST
Supervisor's Office
E6248 US 2
Ironwood, MI 49938
906-932-1330
www.fs.usda.gov/ottawa

PICTURED ROCKS NATIONAL
LAKESHORE
N8391 Sand Point Road
P.O. Box 40
Munising, MI 49862-0040
906-387-2607; **nps.gov/piro**

PIGEON RIVER COUNTRY
FOREST MGT. UNIT
9966 Twin Lakes Road
Vanderbilt, MI 49795
989-983-4101
michigan.gov/dnrpigeonriver

SAULT STE MARIE FIELD OFFICE/
LAKE SUPERIOR STATE FOREST
2001 Ashmun Street
Sault Ste. Marie, MI 49783
906-635-5281

SHINGLETON FIELD OFFICE/
LAKE SUPERIOR STATE FOREST
Box 67, M 28
Shingleton, MI 49884
906-452-6227

SLEEPING BEAR DUNES
NATIONAL LAKESHORE
9922 Front Street
Empire, MI 49630
231-326-5134; **nps.gov/slbe**

TRAVERSE CITY FIELD OFFICE/
PERE MARQUETTE STATE FOREST
North Arbutus Lake Road
Traverse City, MI 49686
231-922-5280

INDEX

● ●

ABOUT THE AUTHOR

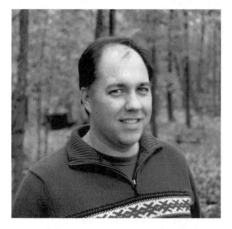

As a native of Michigan, Matt Forster has camped all over the Great Lake State. He's carried his gear in backpacks, Duluth packs, saddlebags, and car trunks and slept in tents, pop-ups, camper vans, and RVs. He and his wife live in Michigan with their two young children, who are both just experiencing camping for the first time. These days, camping trips often come down to tossing the tent in the back of the car, loading up way too much equipment, and praying for good weather (a necessity with two kids in tow).

As a freelance writer, Matt is the author of *Backroads & Byways of Michigan* (The Countryman Press), *Backroads & Byways of Ohio* (The Countryman Press), *Colorado: An Explorer's Guide* (The Countryman Press), *Best Hikes Near Detroit and Ann Arbor* (FalconGuides), and a travel app for Michigan's Grand Traverse region called *Up North! Grand Traverse* (available on iOS and Android devices).

DEAR CUSTOMERS AND FRIENDS,

SUPPORTING YOUR INTEREST IN OUTDOOR ADVENTURE, travel, and an active lifestyle is central to our operations, from the authors we choose to the locations we detail to the way we design our books. Menasha Ridge Press was incorporated in 1982 by a group of veteran outdoorsmen and professional outfitters. For many years now, we've specialized in creating books that benefit the outdoors enthusiast.

Almost immediately, Menasha Ridge Press earned a reputation for revolutionizing outdoors- and travel-guidebook publishing. For such activities as canoeing, kayaking, hiking, backpacking, and mountain biking, we established new standards of quality that transformed the whole genre, resulting in outdoor-recreation guides of great sophistication and solid content. Menasha Ridge continues to be outdoor publishing's greatest innovator.

The folks at Menasha Ridge Press are as at home on a whitewater river or mountain trail as they are editing a manuscript. The books we build for you are the best they can be, because we're responding to your needs. Plus, we use and depend on them ourselves.

We look forward to seeing you on the river or the trail. If you'd like to contact us directly, join in at trekalong.com or visit us at menasharidge .com. We thank you for your interest in our books and the natural world around us all.

SAFE TRAVELS,

BOB SEHLINGER
PUBLISHER